CHRONIC CHILDHOOD DISORDER —
Promoting Patterns of Adjustment

CHRONIC CHILDHOOD DISORDER - Promoting Patterns of Adjustment

IVAN B. PLESS, BA, MD, FAAP, FRCP(C).
Associate Professor of Pediatrics, Preventive Medicine and Community Health, University of Rochester School of Medicine and Dentistry; Director, Children's Habilitation Services, Strong Memorial Hospital; Project Director, Rochester Child Health Studies of Chronically Ill Children.

PHILIP PINKERTON, MB, ChB(Hons), MD, FRC Psych, DPM
Lecturer in Paediatric Psychiatry, University of Liverpool; Consultant Physician in Psychological Medicine, Royal Liverpool Children's Hospital and Alder Hey Children's Hospital; Visiting Consultant, Liverpool Area School Health Service

 Henry Kimpton Publishers   LONDON 1975

© 1975 by Henry Kimpton Publishers
106 Hampstead Road, London NW1

All rights reserved. No part of this publication may be reproduced, stored in a retrieval system, or transmitted, in any form or by any means, electronic, mechanical, photocopying, recording or otherwise, without the prior permission of the publishers.

ISBN 0 85313 791 9

Printed in Great Britain by
Unwin Brothers Limited,
The Gresham Press, Old Woking, Surrey

To the children
and their families
who taught us so much –
especially our own

Contents

FOREWORD Professor J. Tizard	9
FOREWORD Professor R. J. Haggerty	11
PREFACE	13
INTRODUCTION	15
I The Concept of Adjustment	**21**
Disease, disability and handicap	21
Adjustment vs. normality	22
The self-concept model	24
The coping model	27
An integrated model of adjustment	29
A concluding caveat	32
II The Assessment of Adjustment	**34**
Objective measures	36
Subjective measures	40
Projective measures	53
III Long-term Adjustment to Chronic Disorder	**59**
Optimal adjustment in the adult	60
How long is long-term?	63
Consequences during adolescence	64
Consequences during adulthood	72
IV Short-term Adjustment to Chronic Disorder	**87**
General studies of adjustment	89
Scholastic performance as an indirect indicator	95
Psychological maladjustment in specific chronic illnesses	106
Common threads antecedent to maladjustment	162
V Therapeutic Intervention to Promote Adjustment	**168**
Determinants of intervention	168
The strategy of intervention	186
Emergent principles	202
REFERENCES	211
INDEX	241

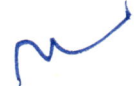

Acknowledgements

Dr Pless gratefully acknowledges the encouragement and support provided by a Milbank Memorial Fund Faculty Fellowship. Much of the research described has also been funded in part by U.S. Public Health Service Grant HS-00467 and by U.S. Public Health Service Research Scientist Career Development Award (HS-47255). Pat Corbett, Marion Repenter and the other members of the Rochester Child Health Study team provided invaluable assistance in the preparation of the references and typing of the manuscript.

Due acknowledgement is made by Dr Pinkerton to the Medical Research Committee of the former United Liverpool Hospitals (Research Scheme No 103) for fostering the clinical research alluded to in this text, His thanks are due too, to Molly Anson and Jeanette Gregg for their painstaking task of typing and retyping the manuscript.

Both authors are indebted to their many paediatric and psychiatric friends and colleagues, on both sides of the Atlantic, for the stimulus of interdisciplinary exchanges so essential to the development of professional insight.

Foreword
by Professor Jack Tizard
Research Professor of Child Development, University of London Institute of Education; Director of the Thomas Coram Research Unit

The authors describe this comprehensive and thoughtful review of problems of chronic childhood disorder as primarily 'an exercise in analysis'. However the literature on physical disability is vast, and extremely scattered, and even to bring it together and order it as has been done here is an exercise in synthesis. And to emphasize principles common to the treatment of children with diseases which are quite different in nature is a further step towards synthesis. Dr Pless and Dr Pinkerton remind us in a very concrete way that 'there is no such thing as sickness, only sick people' whose common human needs are not simply epiphenomenal accompaniments of the handicaps that make them 'sick'. It is the communality of their problems and of how to deal with them which forms the core of the discussion.

Dr Pless and Dr Pinkerton are concerned with psychodynamic and social processes that affect the health and well-being of children and families. Concepts of normality, of self-image, of adjustment, of inferiority, of compensation are central to our understanding of these problems. These are elusive concepts which are in practice difficult or perhaps impossible to measure. In consequence, as the authors point out, many surveys of disabled children have relied almost exclusively upon projective tests and unstandardized ratings; the shortcomings of these are well known, and it is probable that much of the confusion in the literature arises from methodological weaknesses of research rather than from real differences in phenomena. As Dr Pless and Dr Pinkerton show, there is, despite some apparent contradictions, a marked agreement in the findings of many investigators, working more or less in ignorance of each other and concerned with children (and families) whose diagnoses and disabilities are apparently very different.

In a final section the authors bring the findings together and use them to illustrate principles upon which to base practice that will truly promote patterns of adjustment. They emphasize paediatric, psychiatric and family approaches to chronic childhood disorder, and though they say rather little directly about the school and the educational process, they make it clear that the principles they advocate apply as much to education as to paediatrics, social work and child psychiatry. And by widening the focus of attention to include not just the disorder, or indeed just the child, but the child as a developing member of a family and of society they provide a rare insight into the meaning of 'comprehensive' services – services which are enabling rather than simply remedial.

JACK TIZARD

Foreword
by R. J. Haggerty, MD
Professor of Pediatrics, University of Rochester School of
Medicine and Dentistry, Rochester, NY

Pediatrics was founded and developed as a specialty because of the enormous burden acute illness placed on children. At the turn of the century, even in developed countries, one out of ten children did not survive their first birthday largely because of the toll of acute infectious diseases. Most pediatricians active even today were recruited to the field when acute illnesses such as poliomyelitis, meningitis, and diarrhea were the major problems seen in hospitals. Indeed it is likely that most of us were recruited to pediatrics in part because our personalities were most comfortable with patients with short-term illnesses, with acute crises. We enjoyed saving lives and we needed the thanks of the grateful parents of the survivors. What chronic disease there was in hospitals was of less urgency and, therefore, received a lower priority in our training. Much of it was cared for in settings other than where we trained – chronic disease hospitals, doctors' offices, community agencies, or received little attention at all from the medical profession. The situation has now changed.

Chronic disease is today the major health problem of children. Most of us are ill prepared to deal with children who do not get well, with children in whom small progress in improved function is all we can hope for, and with parents of such children who, in having to live daily with the burden, can be forgiven for being less openly grateful to us, for we have done so little for them.

Coming, as it does at this time in the history of the development of child health, this book on chronic illness by a pediatrician and a psychiatrist, who have seen earlier than most the needs of the chronically ill child and his family, is a landmark. It reviews most of what is known about the common psychosocial problems associated with chronic childhood disease. They note the sometimes conflicting and confusing data, and even more distressing the absence of data about many of the most fundamental questions of what causes one child with a disability to function well and another not to.

But the book is not pessimistic. It outlines a comprehensive strategy to approach helping children and their families to function better. It outlines practical steps every physician who deals with these problems can follow and it shows where data exist to guide and where clinical judgment, compassion and good sense must alone suffice.

As pediatrics moves from crisis medicine, to concern for improving functioning, from cure to care, from patch-up to prevention, this synthesis of what is known will be a beacon for all interested in child health to follow. Pediatricians have been late in coming to the philosophy of 'to cure, rarely; to improve function, often; to support and care, always.' This book will help move us toward the day when we can assist all children to reach their full potential, when we and society can accept the handicapped, value their strengths, and not demand that all children be alike and perfect, else we relegate them to places out-of-sight, out-of-mind. This is perhaps the greatest lesson to be learned from this book – tolerance of differences and addition of skills to the physician who wishes to help those who are different lead more effective lives.

R. J. HAGGERTY

Preface

In 1928, Allen and Pearson reported on the emotional problems of the physically handicapped child. Over the succeeding years, many hundred similar reports have appeared, of which a significant and growing proportion are based on rigorously designed and carefully executed scientific studies. No longer can there be any doubt that as a group, children with chronic disorders are more likely to experience psychosocial difficulties than their healthy peers. There is also no doubt that when such difficulties supervene, they frequently prove to be more disabling than the underlying physical disorder.

Despite this formidable array of evidence, remarkably little has been achieved to diminish the frequency of maladjustment among these children or more positively, to promote healthy patterns of adjustment. One explanation is that the observations and findings so far reported have not been sufficiently integrated to allow a course of intervention to be developed. Such a plan needs to be based upon existing knowledge. It must take account of clues provided in the numerous disparate reports of earlier successes and failures. But even more must it take account of the realities involved in the delivery of medical care to children. Variation in communities' resources, in availability of services, in the manner in which physicians are compensated, in their attitudes and training, and in a host of other factors, make any simple formula for action only likely to succeed to a limited extent.

We have aimed this text directly at all physicians and other health professionals who are responsible in any way for the care of these children. Our intention is to assist them in fulfilling this responsibility more effectively by offering practical suggestions. These suggestions are, in turn, based upon an integrated conceptual model of the processes by which maladjustment occurs (and may, hopefully, be prevented) as a consequence of chronic illness in childhood.

I.B.P.

P.P.

Introduction

Children with chronic illness or disability comprise at least 5-10% of the population under the age of 16. In future, that number is likely to increase, so that with declining volume of infectious and nutritional disorders, a progressive proportion of the physician's work must involve the care of these children. Most chronic illness is complex in that successful treatment calls for a high degree of clinical skill coupled with specific technical expertise. The average family doctor or general paediatrician may therefore need to share his management with various particular system specialists.

Yet, over and above the optimum use of drug regimes and appliances it is our belief that some essential elements of care remain lacking. Experienced clinicians share this conviction by recognizing that management is more than simply treating the disease. More attention must be paid to the child as a person to insure that the disease (or its treatment) does not seriously affect developing personality or psychological well-being. This concern has a number of roots.

The sensitive clinician is frequently struck by the extent to which children and their families are as burdened by social and behavioural difficulties as by the direct effects of the disease itself; while psychologists and social workers called upon to treat these difficulties echo this concern. In other words, children with long-term illness seem especially likely to have problems in 'adjustment.'

Used in this context, the term 'adjustment' has two distinct meanings. In one sense, it can mean the extent to which the patient has 'accepted' the reality of his condition and has learned how best to adapt to it, making optimal use of his remaining skills and abilities, coming to terms with functional impairment, and the inevitability of treatment. The second sense conveys the concept of psychological balance or freedom from abnormality in face of pathological circumstances. It is with the latter meaning that we are chiefly concerned, while recognizing that for some patients, psychological well-being is best achieved by refusing to 'accept' the reality of the illness and the disabilities it imposes.

Assessment of the evidence for psychosocial maladjustment as a predictable consequence of chronic illness is one of our major preoccupations. But whether or not the evidence is substantial, when psychological problems are added to basic medical ones, treatment becomes more difficult, successful rehabilitation more problematic, and the ultimate care more costly. If, therefore, emotional sequelae are predictable, and if we can learn how to intervene effectively, there can be no excuse for failing to mount appropriate preventive services; but for whom, when, and in what fashion?

There is no dearth of papers which simply offer speculative opinions, review the findings of others, or draw their conclusions from inadequate clinical experience. Undoubtedly, however, the most reliable 'evidence' upon which to base the provision of special health services derives from properly planned research.

In reviewing the relevant literature, therefore, the main streams of thought will be identified, their supporting framework evaluated, and an attempt made to synthesize salient features emerging from each reported study, in order to achieve some kind of integrated formulation. Not all research endeavours are intended to test specific hypotheses, and in fairness, many make no pretence at scientific rigor. Most of these are essentially descriptive in character but no less valuable if they distil extensive clinical experience. There is scope for both types of approach.

No attempt has been made to cover the entire literature in this area. Much of it is, in any case, repetitious and even more of it of limited value. In a classic monograph first published in 1946, and revised in 1953, Barker and his colleagues critically reviewed more than 800 studies in a singularly comprehensive manner. No subsequent publication has contributed as much to an appreciation of the value — and the short-comings — of

INTRODUCTION   17

research in this field. The authors went beyond simply summarizing the existing literature; they delineated the fundamental model of methodology for future investigators, and thereby established a significant landmark.

This was followed in 1960 by a further important classic published by one of Barker's colleagues, Beatrice Wright. Her book, *Physical Disability — A Psychological Approach,* draws upon 250 studies, but unlike the original report does not adopt a critical or evaluative stance in regard to the research itself. Rather does she synthesize the findings more successfully so that in the end the reader gains a thorough understanding and clearer management directions regarding physical disablement. An unusual feature of the book is the skilful manner in which autobiographical accounts by disabled persons themselves are interwoven with the more objective scientific data. It is in all an immensely readable and human document which still retains its freshness after 15 years.

In the period since the publication of Wright's book, several other contributions have appeared, of considerable merit. Both McDaniel (1969) and Safflios-Rothschild (1970) deal with the problems of chronic illness primarily from a psychological or socio-psychological perspective. Both deal chiefly with adults, while Trapp and Himmelstein (1962), Cruickshank (1963), Kellmer-Pringle (1964), Dinnage (1970, 1972), McMichael (1971), and Pilling (1973) are each broadly based research reviews of chronic illness in childhood.

Special mention must be made of the report of the Carnegie United Kingdom Trust (1964) which provided a detailed account of the problems of 600 handicapped children and their families, that of Rutter, Tizard and Whitmore, (1970), an extensive epidemiological survey that included both physically and mentally handicapped children, and the recent reports of the nationwide studies of the Rand Corporation in the US (Brewer and Kakalik, 1974). During this period, a new edition of Bowley and Gardner's text was published (1972), emphasizing 'educational and psychological guidance.' American books equally oriented toward providing practical advice for the family and physician include Weiner (1973), Debusky and Dombro (1970), Noland (1971) and Downey and Low (1974). Finally, several texts and monographs have been aimed at specific chronic illnesses in childhood, *e.g.* those of Goldin (1971) and Bagley (1971) deal with epilepsy; Roskies (1972) with thalidomide victims; Katz (1970) on haemophilia; Schlesinger and Meadow (1972) on deafness, and Patterson *et al* (1973) on cystic fibrosis.

This spate of publications clearly suggests a growing interest in the problems of the child with a chronic disorder. Taken together, they should permit the development of an integrated model of the processes leading to successful adjustment — applicable to the practicalities of everyday medical care. We share the impatience expressed by so many in recent years — that too much time has elapsed between the results of extensive research reported in so many publications and their implementation. By examining the findings of others and combining them with our own experience, we have attempted in this text to construct a framework for action. We agree, too, that it is not enough to be able to predict 'which children are likely to come off worst,' but that we must be able to intervene effectively. It is clear, that most children 'at risk' need 'more support, more medical attention, more suitable education, more counselling, more care.' (Pringle, 1974). But, in addition to offering *more* help in each of these ways, health workers need guidance in *how* to provide this help and more understanding of the rationale that lies behind the strategies of intervention recommended. It is to this end that we have directed our attention.

This book is divided into five parts. Sections I and II describe the concept of adjustment and the procedures that have been employed to try to measure or assess it. Psychological changes that may result from chronic illness are extensively reviewed together with mechanisms involved.

Sections III and IV examine the evidence for problems of adjustment among the chronically ill and disabled, both in their short-term and long-term consequences, and in respect of their various clinical connotations.

Section V seeks to evaluate the outcome of various therapeutic approaches either aimed at primary prevention or manifest treatment of the established problem.

Finally, on the basis of these accumulated data, an attempt is made to formulate certain broad principles upon which to

INTRODUCTION

base the strategy of individual therapeutic intervention.

In this book we have attempted to integrate the existing body of knowledge, opinion, and experience, from widely dispersed sources. The first step toward a concerted approach must be a conceptual framework which unites existing fragments. The second step is to place that framework within the limitations of an imperfect world in such a way as to enable it to be applied to everyday situations.

1

The Concept of Adjustment

DISEASE, DISABILITY AND HANDICAP

The terms disease, illness and impairment are frequently used interchangeably. In general, the differences are so slight as to be immaterial. When used, however, in place of disability or handicap, the result may be confusing. Table 1 attempts to clarify the meanings intended.

Table 1. **Relationships Between Impairment, Disability and Handicap**

Biological	Behavioural	
	Personal	*Social*
Impairment ⟶	Disability ⟶	Handicap
Synonyms ⌈ Disease ⌉ Illness Defect Disorder ⌊ Condition ⌋	Direct behavioural manifestation of impairment	Effect of disability in performance of specific activities

The distinctions are important both conceptually and semantically. In general, as the figure shows, the terms 'disease, illness, impairment, disorder or condition' are used to describe the pathophysiological process which represents the basic, underlying substrate, *e.g.* diabetes, cerebral palsy, arthritis. 'Disability' is the immediate direct manifestation of disease as it affects behaviour. Thus, the disability produced by arthritis may involve limitation in limb movement, walking with a limp, inability to walk at all, or the presence of pain or swelling. Similarly, the disability experienced by an asthmatic child is manifested as wheezing and shortness of breath during attacks. 'Handicap' is a term that should be reserved for the consequences of disablement in relation to the performance of specific goal-related activities. (It is salutary to remember the use of the term in racing and similar sports in which competitors are equalized by various means.) It refers in fact to the extent to which patients are disadvantaged in the performance of some action. A musician would be severely handicapped if he lost his hearing, an artist if he lost his sight. The notion, however, of generalized handicap imposed by cerebral palsy, epilepsy or comparable chronic illness is unjustified and misleading. Moreover, it has unfortunate psychosocial consequences. Regrettably, the idea of a generally handicapped person (as opposed to one handicapped in some specific area) is deeply rooted in the attitudes of the non-disabled and strongly influences their behaviour toward the disabled. These attitudes and behaviours may equally influence the self-perception of the patient. When the term 'handicapped' is applied to the child rather than to his ability to perform a specific task, there is a tendency for him to see himself as limited in areas unrelated to his illness. The child with spina bifida, for example, unable to walk, may easily become convinced that he is equally incapable of competing scholastically, painting or even appreciating let alone performing music, etc.! This represents the phenomenon of 'spread' (Wright, 1960), *i.e.* a generalized devaluation of body function and perhaps even a devaluation of the 'self' as a person. Semantic precision is therefore of importance in describing this group of problems.

ADJUSTMENT VS. NORMALITY

Despite its central role, and the ease and frequency with which the term is used, the concept of adjustment is a difficult one to translate into objective, measurable terms. Trying to define it is like struggling with the concept of 'normality.' Indeed, conceptually, the two terms are sufficiently similar to make analogous comparisons between them.

According to Offer and Sabshin (1966), for example, the term 'normality' has four different meanings in common usage. The first is the concept of normality as health, or the absence of disease. This is a reasonable rather than an ideal state of function akin to Romano's definition of a healthy person as 'one who is reasonably free of undue pain, discomfort or disability.'

A second view is that of normality as an ideal or Utopian state. This draws on a psychoanalytic view in which the optimal operation of the psychic apparatus and its mental characteristics culminate in optimal functioning. The definition of health suggested by the World Health Organization incorporates this concept — 'Health is a state of complete physical, mental and social well-being and not merely the absence of disease and illness.' In Freud's words, 'Normality is an ideal fiction' or, to paraphrase Rogers, 'The fully functioning person is a platonic ideal, a goal not to be obtained, only to be approximated.'

A third view equates normality with the average: the middle range of the distribution of traits or characteristics in which both extremes are equally deviant and, hence, abnormal. This view is one upon which many psychological tests are based — the assumption being that, as with intelligence, other testable attributes are 'normally distributed' in a population.

Finally, there is a school which views normality as a process — the end result of interacting systems that change over time; a phenomenon always to be viewed from the standpoint of temporal progression. This concept is not exclusive of the others but, rather, an alternative modality along which each of them could be considered.

In the case of adjustment, the problem is further clouded by varying concepts of what is 'good,' 'healthy,' or 'normal'; and by two additional factors peculiar to the situation of disablement. Is it realistic to apply to the disabled the standards applicable where there is no disability? For example, if scholastic progress is taken as one index of adjustment, what allowances should be made for the school loss inevitably stemming from the disability?

Moreover, adjustment frequently refers to the more specific phenomenon of *adaptation* to disability. The assumption is that there are good and bad, or healthy and unhealthy modes of adaptation. It is important to distinguish between this usage — the process of adjustment *to* disability — and the more general sense in which disability may or may not play a part. In most of the studies reviewed, it is global adjustment which is implied. Thus, if the disabled as a group display higher frequency of certain psychologically undesirable behaviours, and all other things are equal, we could conclude that disability plays a contributing role in the pathogenesis of these behaviours. A link can be constructed between these separate concepts by assuming that when, in the process of adaptation, a child adopts unhealthy mechanisms, *e.g.* excessive denial, there exists a predisposition to maladjustment of the more general kind. In the search for evidence to support this assumption, the work of the social psychologists is particularly germane.

THE SELF-CONCEPT MODEL

The somatopsychological relationship between physique and behaviour has been defined by social psychologists (*e.g.* Barker *et al.*, 1953) as 'those variations in physique that affect the psychological situation of a person by influencing the effectiveness of his body as a tool for action, or by serving as a stimulus to himself or others.' This socio-psychological approach provides a clue to a concept of adjustment of relevance to the chronically ill child. Bodily illness can contribute to the formation of self-concept, which, in turn, affects behavioural adjustment (Fig. 1).

Physique or health status is thus seen to contribute to the phenomenal qualities of an individual — the way he perceives himself and is perceived by others — in contrast to his physical or objective properties (his 'noumenal' self, the self as it really is). The extent to which a child's disability intrudes on his 'life space,' *i.e.* obstructs the performance of specific behavioural tasks, also determines how far psychological mechanisms will be brought into play to help cope with the situation. Much of the work of the followers of Kurt Lewin (1936), the field theorist, and, in particular, Meyerson, Wright and Barker, has been devoted to describing these mechanisms and the circumstances under which they are utilized. These investigators point out that the individual with a disability, be he blind or crippled, lives on the border of two worlds, that of the normal and that of the handicapped. The necessary

THE CONCEPT OF ADJUSTMENT

THE SELF-CONCEPT MODEL

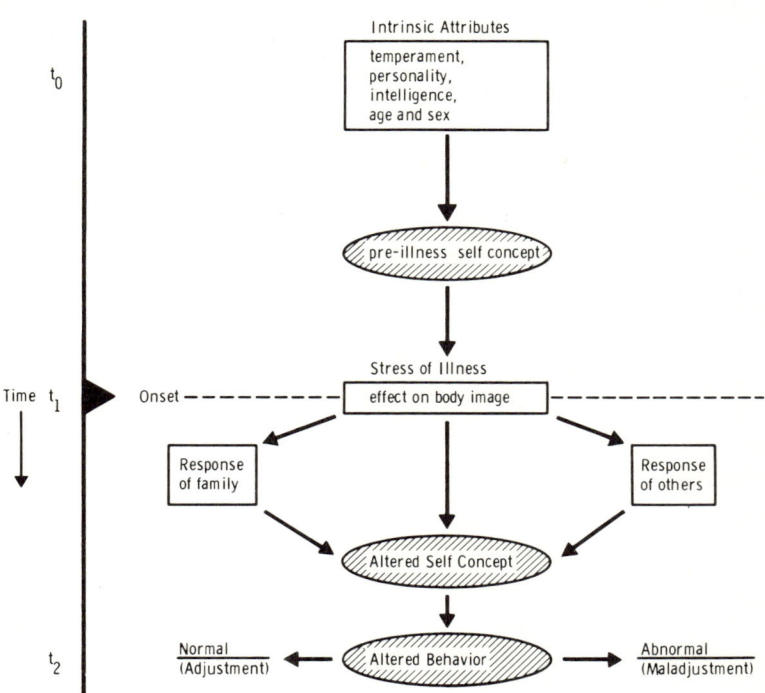

Fig. 1

involvement of the disability in ongoing activity determines the world in which he operates. However, the partial nature of most disablement makes it difficult to predict how far society will accept the handicapped person's own judgment of his abilities. New situations therefore pose a constant challenge and the way in which the disabled react may be equated with psychological adjustment.

Three patterns of reaction are commonly described: withdrawal, rejection (or denial), and acceptance. It is usually assumed that the first two are unhealthy, the third the most desirable. This assumption is, however, a value judgment with a tenuous experimental or empirical basis. If an individual is genuinely happier and functions more effectively when he withdraws from a challenging situation or when he denies the limitations of his disability, he is, at least in one sense, well-adjusted. That is, his self is in harmony with his situation — through a choice of mechanism most appropriate to his personal characteristics.

Another link between this model and adjustment is the extent to which the disabled child's prior encounters with new physical or psychological situations induces a 'set' such that most other new situations are reacted to in similar fashion even though the disability does *not* intervene — the 'spread' phenomenon already attributed to the writings of Beatrice Wright. The constant repetition of such experiences is thought to lead ultimately to devaluation of self-concept.

Healthy persons frequently make judgments of this kind about the handicapped, and the literature on stereotyping contains many other illustrations. Familiar to paediatricians, for example, is the strong inclination by parents to protect a disabled child even in areas totally unrelated to his disability; Green's (1964) 'vulnerable child syndrome' describes a comparable 'spread' following earlier critical illness.

Many investigators, nevertheless, continue to equate 'adjustment' with 'acceptance', or with a variety of compensatory reactions. Thus, Sommers (1944) describing adjustive behaviour in blind adolescents defines it as 'wholesome' in that 'the limitations resulting from the handicap are recognized and accepted and the subject tries to minimize them by substituting for (them). A sound competitive spirit with respect to accessible goals is demonstrated and in discussing problems regarding the handicap, no evasiveness is shown.' In Sommers' terminology, therefore, adjustment means that the subject is able to deal easily with the problems of everyday life. By contrast, a variety of symptoms such as strong self-centredness, emotional instability, intensive worrying and anxiety are cited as signs of maladjustment. Between these two extremes other reactions, such as overcompensation through aggression, denial, or withdrawal, may be found.

Dembo and her co-workers (1956) describe 'adjustment' in

similar terms appropriate to the disabled or chronically ill child. In their paradigm, the question of 'acceptance' remains a pivotal concern, but distinction is made between simple acceptance of the *status quo* and acceptance of one's condition. While it may be greatly inconveniencing or limiting in particular activities, it does not spread to unrelated areas, and, hence, devalue the individual in a global way.

THE COPING MODEL

A second major school of thought equates adjustment to physical illness with the mechanisms used in coping with stress of any kind (Fig. 2).

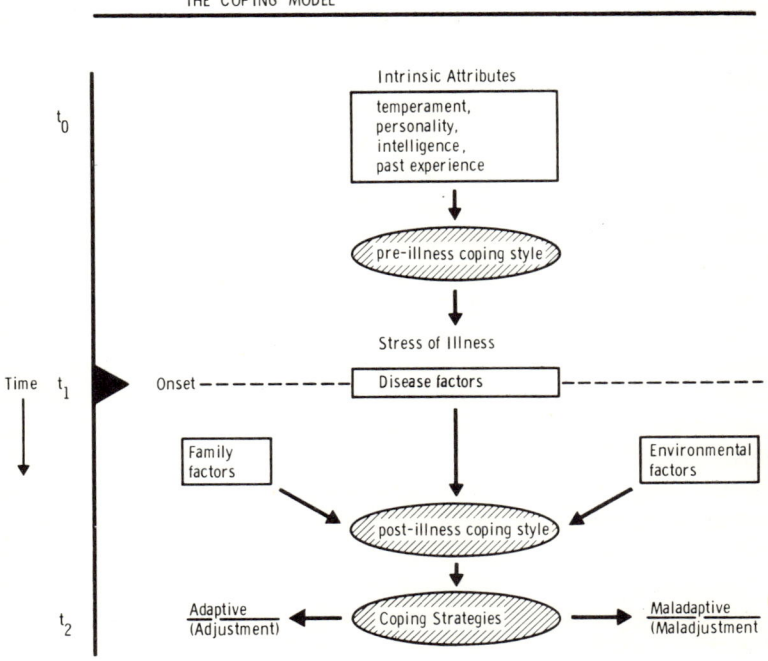

Fig. 2

Lipowski (1970) has offered a conceptual framework for this aspect of illness behaviour. He begins by pointing out that the term 'coping' is itself ambiguous and depends, in part, on the perspective of the definer. Lazarus (1966), for example, views coping as 'the strategies employed for dealing with threat.' The sociological position, on the other hand, views it as the 'instrumental behaviour and problem solving capacities of persons in meeting life demands and goals' (Mechanic, 1968). In Lipowski's model, these apparently opposing views are seen as complementary: physical illness or disability is conceived of as 'a form of psychological stress involving threat of suffering and losses, but *also* as a set of adaptational tasks where success may result in psychological growth.' Thus, Lipowski defines coping as 'all cognitive and motor activities which a sick person employs to preserve his bodily and psychic integrity, to recover reversibly impaired function, and compensate to the limit for any irreversible impairment.'

He also distinguishes between the patient's coping *style* and coping *strategies*. Style refers to 'an enduring disposition to deal with challenges . . . with a specific constellation of techniques.' Strategy involves techniques actually employed by the sick person to deal with his illness and its consequences. Accordingly, strategies represent an expression of both coping style *and* attempts to try new approaches. It is in this latter area that rehabilitative efforts take place. Presumably, success prospects are enhanced if the therapist builds upon an understanding of the patient's coping style.

Depending on how appropriate it is to the child's age and situation, and how effective in reaching the desired goal, the coping process can be thought of as adaptive or maladaptive. Lipowski suggests that the determinants of both style and strategy include *intrapersonal factors,* (such as age, personality, intelligence, the timing of the illness), *disease related* factors, (such as the type of disability, its location, rate of onset, prognosis), and finally, *environmental factors,* (such as social context, *e.g.* the family). He then lists and describes coping styles in two broad categories — cognitive and behavioural.

A similar conceptual model has been developed by Mattsson (1972) to examine the psychosocial adaptation of children with chronic illness. Coping behaviour is interpreted to include 'all the adaptational techniques used by an individual to master a major psychologic threat and its attendant negative feelings in order to allow him to achieve personal and social goals.' Included are the use of cognitive functions, motor activity, emotional expression, and psychologic defenses such that successful coping would result in adaptation, *i.e.* effective functioning. Thus, adjustment is equated with adaptation, and this in turn is conceived of in terms of effective functioning in the home, school, and in relations with peers. This is an easy formulation to accept; the difficulty lies in discovering appropriate measures of 'effective functioning' in each of these areas.

Mattsson suggests several criteria, *i.e.* age—appropriate dependence on the family; little need for secondary gain from the illness; acceptance of both limitations and responsibilities imposed by the illness; and the ability to find satisfaction in a 'variety of compensatory activities and intellectual pursuits.' He suggests, in addition, that cognitive flexibility, the appropriate release and control of emotions, and the adaptive use of psychologic defenses (*e.g.* denial, isolation, and identification) are each components in successful adaptation. These ideas are based upon extensive review of the literature as well as Mattsson's own considerable field experience. The references he cites, however, are predominantly drawn from psychiatric studies on relatively small groups of patients. It is, nevertheless, a reasonable formulation warranting testing on a wider scale.

AN INTEGRATED MODEL OF ADJUSTMENT

So far, in relation to chronic childhood illness, the process of adjustment (or maladjustment) has usually been construed as either stemming from the impact of illness on the child's self-concept, or from breakdown in the coping process, engendered by the implications of the lesion or the reactions of others. However, through our own work, and in reviewing the work of others, we have become increasingly aware that neither 'model' taken alone can do full justice to the complexities involved.

Partly this is because the process is not a static one; it extends through childhood into adult life, with ultimate stabilization as arguably its most important end-product. But adult functioning itself has multiple determinants, most of them interrelated, so that overall, the picture is exceptionally complex.

The integrated model portrayed in Fig. 3 attempts to illustrate some of these complexities; first by demonstrating how coping and self-concept, the two earlier models, may themselves be linked — possibly as differing manifestations of the same phenomenon — and secondly, by suggesting cybernetic circuits between family attitudes, other social factors, the child's own basic attributes and his response to illness. Based on evidence that the process is dynamic, a series of 'feed-back' loops are postulated, of which only two are illustrated. Adjustment changes over time, in that current functioning influences the response of others, which in turn, reciprocally influences future functioning.

Without prejudice to the nature-nurture controversy, the model suggests that many of the child's intrinsic attributes (temperament, personality, intelligence, etc.) are influenced at least in part, by genetic and other familial factors, as well as by social factors outside the family. These attributes in turn determine self-concept and coping style; so that efforts to predict the response to stress engendered by chronic illness must take cognizance of the pre-morbid profile.

The response is no less influenced however, by the nature of the lesion (see p.168), and by the manner in which family, peers, teachers, and 'significant others', react'. Partly these are reactions to the disorder *per se,* but additionally, they are reactions to the behaviour of the child in relation to his illness.

As time progresses, successive cycles of these major determinants (of coping and self-concept) will evolve; so that, at any given point, adjustment or maladjustment, in terms of psychological functioning, will reflect the net product of earlier cycles.

In the sections which follow, evidence will be subsumed to support the view that functioning in early childhood is at least partly predictive of later functioning during adolescence and adult life.

THE CONCEPT OF ADJUSTMENT

AN INTEGRATED MODEL OF ADJUSTMENT

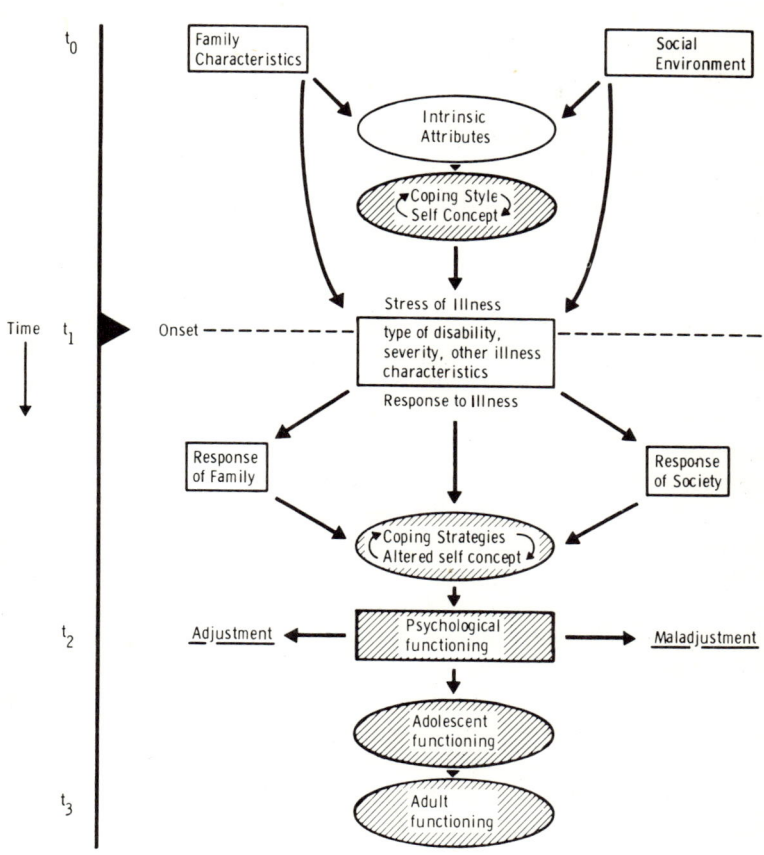

Fig. 3

This composite model, by integrating the role of self-concept with coping mechanisms, provides a strategic basis for therapeutic intervention. Clearly, the earlier that intervention, the greater the opportunity to promote effective adjustment, and thereby prevent maladjustment. But even if maladjustment has already become manifest, the model is still of value in helping to determine which of the many contributing factors may be most amenable to successful therapy.

A CONCLUDING CAVEAT

The very notion of 'adjustment' to an illness is itself ambiguous. One assumption is that where an association can be demonstrated between chronic physical disorder in childhood and various maladjustive psychosocial manifestations, the maladjustment is a consequence of the physical disorder. Clearly, if it could be shown that children were free of emotional problems prior to the onset of physical illness, and that these problems followed the illness with some regularity, the evidence for a causal relationship would be fairly convincing. If, furthermore, emotional and social problems could be shown to follow more frequently in these chronically ill children than in healthy controls, the case would be virtually unshakable. However, the ideal 'experimental' design needed to produce such conclusive evidence is so very difficult to set up that compromise is necessary. In practice, evidence is more likely to accumulate from a variety of studies each approximating to the ideal in certain respects.

We are therefore interested in two hypotheses. The first, that there is indeed a significant relationship between maladjustment and chronic illness in children; the second, that this relationship is a causal one. 'Significant' in this context is meant incidentally in both its statistical sense and in the common sense — as meaningful in everyday life. For the clinician, the latter sense is what he finds more pertinent.

Among the sources of evidence examined, Section V looks at attempts at prevention or therapeutic intervention. In the long run, such evidence could prove the most convincing. Proof that a problem exists and even clear evidence of its underlying mechanisms is a far cry from demonstrating that something can be done about it. However, the more successful any programme of intervention, based specifically upon the hypothesis that maladjustment is a consequence of physical disorder, the stronger the evidence, albeit indirect, in support of that hypothesis.

Accordingly, throughout this text, chief emphasis is laid on the assumption that somatic illness precedes those forms of psychological disturbance judged to represent 'maladjustment'. We fully appreciate that opposing views exist; that emotional stress may trigger, exacerbate or even be a primary factor in the genesis of at least some chronic physical childhood disorders; or that there may even exist a common, possibly genetic substrate, simultaneously responsible for both physical and psychological illness. However, we have chosen, perhaps arbitrarily, to confine our focus to the evidence for a presumed somato-psychic sequence, because it is in the management of this type of problem that we are particularly concerned to alert the clinician in the care of these children.

II

The Assessment of Adjustment

Attempting to establish an operational concept of adjustment in relation to chronic illness clearly poses difficulties. Predictably, therefore, little unanimity has emerged in the choice of method adopted in assessment studies. The wide range of procedures that have in fact been used, reflect both practical and theoretical considerations. Researchers who believe that only overt behaviour is pertinent, place little value in the 'paper and pencil' type of subjective measure. Conversely, those interested in the underlying determinants of behaviour will prefer techniques designed to probe beneath the conscious awareness of the child. This cannot be done with subjective tests.

At the practical level, it may prove uneconomic to have a psychiatric interview with each subject so that proxy tests may be the only practical alternative. It is hardly surprising, therefore, that over the past fifty years no consensus has emerged which favoured one type of approach over another, far less any preference for a single specific measure. Rating scales, inventories and tests have been introduced, become popular and then gradually faded out. The only enduring instruments to stand the test of time are some of the projective measures, notably the figure drawings, the Rorschach, and the TAT or CAT. Over the past 10-15 years various measures of self-ideal discrepancy have enjoyed more popularity and have tended to replace the older all-purpose personality inventories. Apart from this, few genuine developments are discernible.

Generally speaking, the assessment of adjustment can be divided into two broad categories — direct and indirect. *Direct* measures attempt to assess adjustment specifically through objective, subjective or projective techniques.

Indirect procedures are not, in fact, 'measures' in the true sense of the word. They should be viewed more properly as rough indices through which to infer the operation of maladjustment. The most directly relevant of these is evidence that the child has warranted psychiatric treatment. This is *de facto* evidence of maladjustment — whether or not attributable to his physical disability, is another matter. If anything, psychiatric treatment rates in a group of children with chronic illness are likely to be underestimates of the true prevalence of maladjustment because of inadequate psychiatric facilities.

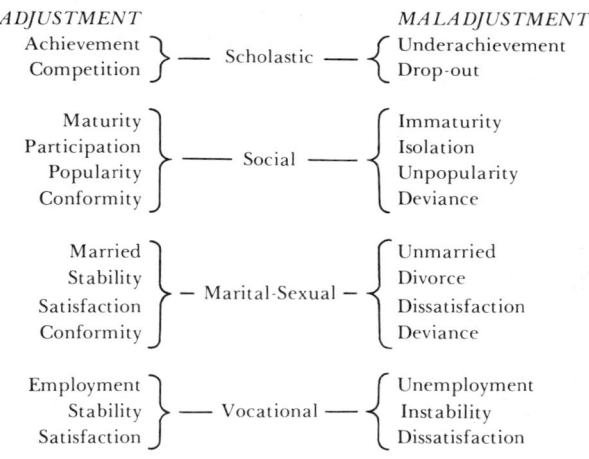

Table 2. **Some Indirect Indicators of Maladjustment**

Other *indirect* indices include academic under-achievement, delinquency, truancy, or extreme social isolation (Table 2). Their counterpart in adult life — criminality, unemployment, marital failure, prolonged bachelorhood or spinsterhood, alcoholism, inappropriate vocational training — each may be regarded as evidence for maladjustment provided their frequency exceeds the incidence in a matched group or in a normative population. Because each of these indirect measures can result from factors other than the presence of chronic illness, the proper comparative conditions must be met before conclusions are drawn. An example is provided by Stearns (1959) in his report of self-destructive behaviour in young diabetic patients. Four cases are described, but although well-documented, the evidence for suicidal tendencies being more frequent among diabetics is inconclusive since no comparison data is reported.

Equivalent reservations apply to direct measures. Because they can be administered at will, however, in contrast to the natural course which governs indirect behaviour, methodological prospects are more encouraging (Weiner and Goldberg, 1974). Literally hundreds of tests and measures of personality and adjustment have been developed for use with children. Most are described and evaluated critically in periodic inventories such as the Mental Measurement Yearbook (Buros, 1972) or Personality Tests and Measures (Buros, 1971). Those we describe are limited to the instruments used in actual studies of children with chronic illnesses. They are summarized in Tables 3, 4 and 5.

OBJECTIVE MEASURES

Observations

The only *completely* objective measures are those based on *direct* observations of behaviour. This is so difficult to achieve that most often the relation between observed behaviour and adjustment has to be inferred indirectly. Schoggen (1974) has made one of the very few attempts to examine psychological and situational factors which could account for differences in behaviour in the physically disabled. The basic data for his study consisted of 'specimen records of behaviour and situation.' Trained observers watched children for sample periods up to 30 minutes, making notes on their behaviour and on the important features of the environment. These observations were made through a special face-mask microphone and battery-powered tape recorder. Seven pairs of children were observed, both at home and at school during free-time activities. Particular attention was paid to social actions directed by environmental agents toward the child subject.

A less structured example of direct observations used to infer progress toward adjustment is provided by Mattsson and Gross (1966). Their studies were based upon children and adolescents with haemophilia. They took advantage of the child's frequent hospital admissions to observe his behaviour toward ward personnel, other patients, and reactions to therapy. A similar approach was used by Reynell (1965) in her study of post-operative disturbances in cerebral palsied children.

Table 3. **Measures to assess psychological adjustment of disabled children**

A. *OBJECTIVE MEASURES*

I. *Behavioural Observations*
Field studies (Schoggen, 1974)
Ward studies (Mattsson, 1966)

II. *Behaviour Ratings* (Parent)
Children's Service Questionnaire
(Kearsley and Snider, 1964)
Child Behaviour Inventory
(Lapouse and Monk, 1958)
Child Scale A
(Rutter and Graham, 1970)

III. *Behaviour Ratings* (Teacher)
Bristol Social Adjustment Guide
(Stott, 1966)
Behaviour Rating Scale
(Cowen, 1970)
Behaviour Rating Checklist
(Quay and Peterson, 1967)
Child Scale B
(Rutter and Graham, 1970)

IV. *Sociometric Ratings*
A Class Play
(Bower, 1962)

V. *Other Measures*
Vineland Social Maturity Scale
(Doll, 1956)

If sufficient such observations could be made in a variety of situations (at home, school and play) without influencing behaviour through the presence of the observer, their importance could prove inestimable. Unfortunately, these conditions are rarely possible. They are expensive and time-consuming, they require highly skilled observers, and the results are sometimes difficult to interpret. In institutional settings, such as schools, observing the frequency of particular behaviours forms the basis for 'learning theory' or 'behavioural modification' techniques. To date, however, this procedure has enjoyed limited potential as a basic investigative tool.

Parent rating scales
Aside from the use of specially trained personnel, there is no shortage of less skilled proxy observers of children's behaviour. The most popular are the child's parents themselves and behavioural rating scales based on parental observations are in fact legion. The frequency with which parents report the presence of symptomatic disturbance in their children is significantly related to the presence of psychological illness as independently determined; that much is well established. Parental bias must always be taken into account, but if the reporting form is properly structured, if it is carefully administered, and in particular if norms have been established for age and sex and sex of parent making the observation, these biases can be minimized. Although students of behaviour continue to debate the validity of self-administered questionnaires, they cannot be discounted pragmatically.

Kearsley et al. (1946) describe one such measure based on 'the parents' perception of the degree to which 49 descriptive characteristics currently applied to their child.' These responses have been standardized by age and sex, and the procedure used in an epidemiological study of children with chronic illnesses (Pless and Roghmann 1971).

Sultz et al. (1972) in studies of children with illness thought to have a psychosomatic origin (p.147), employed a similar procedure based on the work of Lapouse and Monk (1958). Their behavioural inventory was standardized by questioning the parents of 482 children aged between 6 and 12 years to establish the incidence of various behaviours common in this age range.

A similar procedure was devised by Rutter et al. (1970b) for their studies on the Isle of Wight. They evoked parallel forms for use by parents (Child Scale A) and teachers (Child Scale B). The behaviours so listed made it possible to divide children into three principal groups on the basis of their deviant scores — neurotic, aggressive or mixed neurotic and agressive. Although there was little concordance between parental ratings and teacher ratings, when taken together they served to screen out a high proportion of children judged by independent psychiatric assessment to have significant disturbance. These measures were also used in the same study to determine the frequency of behavioural disturbance among children with chronic physical illnesses and to compare these rates with frequency among healthy 'controls'.

Teacher rating scales

Perhaps the most popular form of behavioural assessment using objective measures of this kind are those based upon teacher rating scales. Again the possibility of bias must be acknowledged. For example, teachers are more likely to identify children with disorderly, aggressive behaviour than those who are withdrawn. Nevertheless, with due attention to this bias, a number of scales have been developed and used in studies of adjustment in children with physical illnesses.

Stott's Bristol Social Adjustment Guide (1966), for example, is widely used in Britain for this purpose. Its most extensive application was by Davie, et al. (1972) in their study of the National Cohort of 1958 births. It has also been employed by Williams (1970) in assessing maladjustment in deaf children, and by many others.

In a more complex study of deaf children, Reivich and Rothrock (1972) used the Quay and Peterson Behaviour Problem Checklist (1967). This procedure also makes use of teacher's observations, although it may equally be employed with parents, ward personnel, and clinicians. Through factor analysis, it will identify conduct disorder, personality disorder, and general inadequacy-immaturity dimensions. In the study with deaf children and adolescents, two additional factors — isolation and communication problems — were also noted.

Cowen and his colleagues describe the use of a teacher behaviour rating scale in their studies of children with visual and auditory handicaps (1961), and in their assessment of 'vulnerable children' detected in the early school years (1973). This 17-item scale yields total and overall adjustment scores of proven predictive value in children later diagnosed with psychiatric disturbance, but it must be supported by other adjustment and behavioural measures.

Peer ratings

In addition to parent and teacher ratings of children's

behaviour, it is sometimes possible to obtain the assessment of the child's peers. Although not often feasible (and not without some ethical hazards), such assessments are of considerable value not only in determining adjustment, but in illuminating the social psychology of childhood disability.

The Class Play is part of a set of procedures developed by Bower and Lambert (1962) to help with early identification of emotionally handicapped children in the classroom. It is a two-part sociometric test which requires that children nominate one or more peers for each of 20 roles — half positive and half negative — for an imagined play. In the second part, 30 multiple choice sets of four roles are presented to each child — two roles are positive and two negative. The child is asked to select, for each set, which of the four roles he, his teacher, or his peers consider him best suited for. This procedure formed part of the test battery used in the Rochester studies of children with chronic illnesses.

A similar, but more traditional sociometric procedure was used by Marge (1966) in a study of social status among children with speech handicaps. All children in the class were asked to name three others with whom they would like to work or study; three whom they would like to have in their team for playground games; three whom they would like to take home for dinner; and three whom they would like to have speak for them all day in school, at play, and at home 'if you had a sore throat and could not talk.'

SUBJECTIVE MEASURES

In general, objective measures of the kind so far described are valuable indices of adjustment. They reflect the child's behaviour in the eyes of others but unlike subjective measures tell only indirectly what he thinks about himself. These two parameters, however, are not necessarily interchangeable, and indeed, in a study by Werdelin (1969), although teacher and peer ratings were found to correlate closely, self-ratings were unrelated to either.

In contrast, Cowen and his colleagues (1970) have shown significant correlations between certain parent measures and both peer measures and self-ratings. More of the correlations were significant for girls than boys from which the authors conclude that 'for boys, what is entirely acceptable behaviour at home, may not be acceptable in the schools, and vice versa.' Similarly, Horowitz (1962) has demonstrated that significant relationships exist between anxiety in fourth, fifth and sixth grade children, as assessed by the Children's Manifest Anxiety Scale, a self-concept measure (assessed by Lipsett's scale), and a ranking sociometric measure. Both anxiety and self-concept and anxiety and sociometric status showed consistent negative correlations (high anxiety with low self-concept).

Taken together these findings suggest there is indeed some overlap between objective measures and the subjective scales now to be described. It has been argued that although less sensitive, objective measures, based as they are upon more overt manifestations of maladjustment, are probably more valid and therefore more important indices of disturbance from a social viewpoint. By this criterion, if a child is not sufficiently disturbed to attract outside concern, then professional attention is hardly indicated. The converse argument based upon preventive orientation is that it is more important to identify children before their disturbance becomes overt enough to create concern among parents and teachers.

Table 4. **Measures to assess psychological adjustment of disabled children**

B. *SUBJECTIVE MEASURES*
  I. *Personality Inventories*
     California Test of Personality
        (Thorpe, 1953)
     Brown Personality Inventory
        (Brown, 1934)
     Junior Eysenck Personality Scale
        (Eysenck, 1965)
     Children's Personality Questionnaire
        (Cattell, 1962)
  II. *Anxiety Scales*
     Children's Manifest Anxiety Scale
        (Castaneda, 1956)
     Test Anxiety Scale for Children
        (Sarason, 1958)

III. *Self-Concept Scales*
   Self-Concept Scale
      (Lipsett, 1958)
   Children's Self-Concept Scale
      (Piers & Harris, 1964)
   Self-Concept Inventory
      (Sears, 1971)
   Self-Esteem Inventory
      (Coopersmith, 1959)
   Tell About Yourself
      (Bower, 1960)
   Self-Ideal Q-Sort
      (Cowen, 1973)
IV. *Other Measures*
   Colvin Silhouette Test
      (Colvin, 1964)
   Semantic Differential
      (Osgood, 1957)
   Mood Adjective Check Lists
      (Nowlis, 1956)
   Self-Social Constructs Test
      (Long and Henderson, 1967)

Personality inventories

Subjective measures of the kind shown in Table 4 are even more numerous than parent and teacher rating scales. The first type of test in this category is the personality inventory. The Junior Eysenck Personality Inventory (EPI) is a good example. As with other such measures, the technique is based upon questionnaires in which the answers are limited often to yes or no, or to simple scales of a Likert nature. The EPI (Eysenck, 1965) is designed for use by children between the ages of 7 and 16 and yields data to assess two dimensions of personality — neuroticism and extroversion. It is well standardized and widely used, particularly in Britain. It consists of 108 items.

A more ambitious measure has been used extensively in America since its introduction (Thorpe *et al.* 1953). The California Test of Personality contains two subtests — Personal Adjustment (PA) and Social Adjustment (SA). The sum of the two gives a single score to indicate the child's total adjustment (TA). Its validity has been well established, first by the authors and subsequently by others. In 1958, Smith compared its concurrent validity, *i.e.* the extent to which test scores correspond to measures of concurrent criterion performance (or status) with those of the Rozenzweig Picture-Frustration Study and the Rogers Test of Personality Adjustment. In each case the criterion comprised teacher nominations of very well adjusted and very poorly adjusted children and peer nominations. Smith concluded that 'none of the tests discriminates well enough to be used as a selection instrument for maladjusted pupils in the usual classroom . . . (but) . . . well enough to adjustment status to warrant their use in research.'

Other investigators have reached similar conclusions. Hanlon et al. (1954) found the California test scores to be highly correlated with self-ideal congruence as assessed by the Q-sort techniques. This finding is important because it means that the California could be used to evaluate the success of psychotherapy in improving adjustment. Even before the 1953 revision, the CTP was being used to study the effect of physical illness on psychological adjustment. One of the earliest reports of such use is by Seidenfeld (1948) in his study of 110 children with poliomyelitis. This study failed to show any significant differences in the scores of these children which would indicate maladjustment and the author concluded, 'The standard variety of paper-pencil exploratory questionnaires seems unlikely to lead us very far in ascertaining the basic problems of children with chronic illnesses and disability.' He attributes this pessimism to the ability of the children to 'discern socially acceptable answers' in such tests. (The findings of Kammerer (1940) and of Gates (1946), both equally negative, are cited in support).

The revised form of the CTP is no doubt still susceptible to social desirability responses but has been improved in several other aspects. It consists of 144 questions requiring either a yes or no response, each of which is scored as correct or incorrect. The CTP has been extensively studied and widely described as to how appropriate a measure of adjustment it is. One study has explored the relationship between self-acceptance and adjustment, using the California as a 'rough, external measure of adjustment' largely for its practical aspects (Taylor and Combs, 1952), *i.e.* it is relatively simple to administer and score, and teachers are familiar with measures of this kind.

The results confirmed the hypothesized relation which further validates that it is indeed 'adjustment' that is being measured. (One interesting observation was made by the authors in discussing their findings: since most personality inventories are based upon the individual's making or accepting statements about himself, many of which are derogatory, the well-adjusted might be thought more likely to acknowledge the more critical statements.) The instrument seems robust and flexible and has been used, apparently with success, with deaf children (ages 9-17) (Vegely and Elliott, 1968), and even with the retarded, albeit less successfully (Gardner, 1967).

A more sophisticated measure is the Children's Personality Questionnaire designed by Porter and Cattell (1959). It includes a large number of questions which, after factor analysis, are thought to identify 14 distinct dimensions of personality. These dimensions are each described in bipolar terms, *e.g.* stiff, aloof vs. warm, sociable; emotionally immature, unstable vs. mature, calm, etc. Thus, a comprehensive personality description is built up and can be quantified. Profiles for clinical groups such as neurotics and psychopaths are suggested, although no specific designation of adjustment as such is offered. It has been used by Purcell *et al.* (1969) in a comparison of subgroups of children with asthma.

Anxiety scales

The children's form of the Manifest Anxiety Scale designed originally by Taylor (1953) and modified for use in children by Castaneda *et al.* (1956) has been used extensively in many studies of adjustment in children with physical handicaps. A short form of the scale has been described by Levy (1958) which, in spite of its high correlation with full scale scores, is less frequently cited. A similar measure for use with children is Sarason's Test Anxiety Scale (1958). Attempts have been made with varying degrees of success to adapt these scales for use with the blind (Hardy, 1968).

The great interest in measures for assessing anxiety is based upon the observation that 'anxiety states are among the most common forms of personal disturbance with which clinicians must deal.' Apart from their obvious clinical importance, they relate strongly to other measures of adjustment and self-concept. Thus, they may be used as indirect and approximate measures of adjustment, or may, more properly, be used to modify and aid in the interpretation of other test results, potentially compromised through high anxiety levels during the test administration.

Self-concept scales

At the heart of any formulation that chronic illness may lead to a higher frequency of psychological maladjustment lie assumptions about the effect of the illness on the disabled person's perception of himself. One approach has been to emphasize the actual image a person has of his body; another seeks to gain descriptions of self-concept. It has been asserted that 'the concept of self-evaluation is crucial to an understanding of the role of body image, discrimination, or any other psychological process in disabled children.' (Downing et al. 1961). This is a sweeping statement but we tend to agree with it. If there were entirely satisfactory measures of self-concept or a 'perfect' means for estimating self-evaluation, clinicians and investigators both would have a tool as central to their armamentarium as the stethoscope to the physician.

The notion of body-image has been studied extensively by Fisher and his co-workers, particularly in relation to personality (Fisher and Cleveland, 1958). In their work, they use the term to 'designate the attitudinal framework which defines the individual's long-term concept of his body and also influences his perception of it.' Most of Fisher's work and that of his successors is based upon the pioneering studies of Schilder (1950) who defined the image of the human body simply as 'the picture of our own body which we form in our mind, that is to say the way in which the body appears to ourselves.'

A number of ingenious techniques have been derived to explore this phenomenon, particularly in relation to obesity. For example, Cappon and Banks (1968) used full-length body mirrors and asked nude obese subjects and normal controls to estimate in darkened rooms the width and thickness of their bodies. Glucksman and Hirsch (1969) have an even more complex procedure involving special projections of slides of the body to demonstrate that obese subjects consistently overestimate their own body size both during and following weight loss, whereas no obese subjects underestimate their body size.

Using a questionnaire designed by Secord and Jourard (1953) for measuring 'body cathexis', and a body-image test consisting of 50 items describing body parts and functioning which the respondent rates in terms of positive or negative feelings, Schwab and Harmeling (1968) showed lower body-image scores among psychiatric patients than among the healthy. They also showed that negative feelings about the body were not restricted to parts and functions affected by illness, but extended toward the body as a whole. Among these patients, negative feelings were correlated with indices of emotional distress. Gunderson (1965) has similarly shown an association between actual body size and self-evaluation as assessed by the body-cathexis questionnaire.

The pertinence of these interrelated concepts to the assessment of adjustment is summarized in Gunderson's words as follows: 'In all major personality theories, evaluative attitudes toward body and self have been emphasized as important influences in behaviour.' Psychoanalytically-oriented theorists have postulated the vital role of ego defense mechanisms (Freud, 1946) and 'security operations' (Sullivan, 1954), in maintaining a favourable self-image, and Rogers (1951) has placed self-evaluation at the centre of his theory of personality development and change. Wylie (1961) has documented the importance of 'self-concept' in personality and behavioural research.

Fisher and Cleveland (1958) have amassed convincing evidence concerning the significant part that 'body-image' plays in personality functioning. These investigators go on to report the findings of an elaborate study which convincingly correlates self-evaluation in young, healthy men with biographical information reflecting past experiences at home and school. (Other assertions about the relation between childhood experiences and adjustment in later life will be reviewed in a subsequent section). The studies of Kaplan (1969, 1970) are equally relevant, however, in their demonstration of relationships between self-derogation and

THE ASSESSMENT OF ADJUSTMENT

psychosocial adjustment (measured by self-reports of psychological symptoms, scores on a depressive affect scale, and reports of utilization of psychiatry and other medical resources).

Admittedly, most of the work just described pertains to adults. Both the positiveness of self-concept and the ability to describe it are a function of age (Hess and Bradshaw, 1970). In a study using a modification of the Q-sort technique developed by Stephenson (1953), it has been shown that this construct — a child's perception of himself — is a central factor influencing his behaviour and that congruence between actual and ideal self increases with age, especially in girls (Perkins, 1958). In this application of the Q-sort, children were presented with a stratified random sample of 50 self-referrent statements (*e.g.* 'I am a leader') and instructed to arrange them in order according to the extent to which they were 'like me' or 'unlike me'.

In their studies of the blind and deaf, Underberg (1961) and Bobrove (1964) respectively used modifications of this technique to assess self-ideal discrepancies. The child is asked to sort the statements and then to rank them a second time according to the order in which they would appear for an 'ideal' person. In spite of its sensitivity and reliability, it is unlikely that children younger than the age of 10 are able to use this particular procedure meaningfully. Hanlon and his co-workers (1954) showed that a modified self-ideal Q-sort could, however, be used with adolescents (ages 14-18), and demonstrated that the relation between the two self-concept constructs tends to be positive and normally distributed. They also showed a positive and highly significant relationship with the measure of total adjustment derived from the California Test of Personality.

Similarly, the self-concepts of adolescents during psychiatric hospitalization, as assessed by the Q-sort technique, were significantly more negative than those of 20 similarly aged 'normals', and changes occurred with therapy in the direction predicted (Harrow *et al.* 1968).

The Q-sort is most often used for assessing self-evaluation by examining the discrepancy between ratings of oneself 'as he really thinks he is' and ratings of 'how he would really like to be.' Such discrepancies are thought to reflect the degree of dissatisfaction with oneself. Is such an approach more useful than a direct assessment of self-concept? In an effort to answer this question, Lipsett (1958) devised a self-concept scale using 22 trait-descriptive adjectives prefacing each by the phrase 'I am . . .,' and following each with a 5-point Likert-type rating scale (*i.e.* 'Not at all, Not very often, Some of the time, Most of the time, and All of the time'.) The total score for self-concept was obtained by summing the ratings for each item in a way such that lower scores reflected the degree of self disparagement. A parallel 'ideal-self' scale was created using the same adjectives prefaced by 'I would like to be . . .' The discrepancy score was the subtraction of the total self-concept score from the total self-ideal score. Both scales were administered to approximately 300 fourth, fifth, and sixth grade children on the same day along with the CMAS, and the procedure repeated two weeks later. The results indicated that in spite of high test-retest reliabilities on both measures, and a consistent and significant correlation between anxiety scale scores and discrepancy scores for all but the fifth and sixth grade boys, the negative correlations between anxiety scale scores were consistently higher for both sexes and at all grade levels. Accordingly, Lipsett's Self-concept Scale has won an established place among children's self-evaluation measures although it has not been used often in studies of the handicapped.

A similar but apparently improved measure of self-concept measurement for children was introduced by Piers and Harris in 1964 and has been used in several studies of the chronically ill (Pless, 1975, Korsch *et al.*, 1973). It too is based upon Rogers' self-theory position that adjustment is in part 'a function of self-concept and self-acceptance.' In contrast to Lipsett's measure, this scale has been standardized on children ranging from third grade to tenth grade and has been shown to have satisfactory internal consistency, test-retest reliability, and to be independent of sex and IQ. It was developed from a pool of statements obtained in 1952 by Jersild from children who were asked to describe what they liked and disliked about themselves. After preliminary testing, the original pool of 164 statements were reduced to 80 answerable by 'yes' or 'no,' *e.g.*

'I am a happy person'. The validity of the scale was established by comparing scores of retarded children with the non-retarded. Factor analysis identified six significant factors — behaviour, intellect and school status, physical appearance and attributes, anxiety, popularity, happiness and satisfaction (Piers, 1969).

A similar procedure was developed in 1959 by Coopersmith for use with slightly older children. The Self-esteem Inventory is based upon items selected from the original Rogers and Dymond scale (1954), reworded for use with children. Five psychologists sorted the items into those indicative of high self-esteem and low self-esteem respectively and the resulting questions were tested for comprehensibility. The final measure consists of 50 items which the child is instructed to check as to whether they are 'like me' or 'unlike me'. To validate the scores so obtained, a self-esteem behaviour rating form was created for the children's teachers and principals, which, with the scores on the Iowa Achievement Test, a sociogram, the SMAS, a measure of achievement motivation, and a measure of ideal-self, were all then compared. The Inventory scores were significantly related to academic and social 'success' as estimated by the Achievement test scores and the sociogram. They were also related to the teachers' ratings and the manifest anxiety scores in the expected fashion.

The importance of this measure is that it is clearly related to behavioural expressions. Children 'who had more success experiences were significantly higher in their self-evaluation than those with fewer such experiences.' Unfortunately, to date, the Rochester studies have shown that the form of the responses, involving as they do occasional double negatives, is frequently confusing especially for younger children. Nevertheless, the SEI has been used in a number of studies of children with chronic illnesses and found to be a sensitive and reliable measure of adjustment. In spite of its general acceptability, Coopersmith cautions that 'at the present state of psychological knowledge, a combination of subjective and observer evaluations, taken in conjunction with a constellation of variables . . .' is needed to avoid the pitfalls attendant to the use of any one method separately.

Other measures of a similar kind employed in studies of the

adjustment of children with chronic disorder, include the Self-concept Inventory (Sears, 1971) and the self measures designed by Bower (1960) (A Self Test and Tell About Yourself) for promoting early identification of children with emotional disorders within the school.

Other measures
A number of other measures have been introduced in this sphere which are so novel as to defy classification under any of the previous headings. One such is the Colvin Silhouette Test of Self-concept and Interpersonal Relations (1964) (employed by Garlinghouse and Sharp in their study of the haemophilic child's self-concept in relation to bleeding episodes (1968)). The test is administered by asking the child to point to the one silhouette of a group of 36, all of equal height and appearance, which represents himself in relation to each of 13 operationally-defined dimensions.

Another is the Mood Adjective Check List, developed initially by Nowlis (1956) and adapted for use with children by Hahn and Clark (1967) for their study of the psychophysiological reactivity of children with asthma. The test uses five groups of adjectives to describe anger, tension, depression, bewilderment and positive attitudes — a total of 30 adjectives — which the child is asked to check on a 4-point scale according to the extent to which the adjective reflects his feelings.

In 1957 Osgood and his colleagues introduced the use of the semantic differential technique to study the cognitive meaning or structures of various concepts or ideas. The rationale 'is that words represent things as a mediation process. The meaning which individuals ascribe to the words, or signs, will vary to the extent that their experience with the word or sign varies . . .' The responses have been used to differentiate between disturbed and normal populations by assuming that individual maladjustment will be mirrored on the semantic differential by a tendency to use extremes in checking the scales, by self-ideal discrepancies, or by close relationships between self-concepts and various sickness concepts. The instrument has been widely used because of its flexibility as a research tool, primarily with adults, but on occasion too in the study of disabled children.

One such attempt is described by Downing *et al.* (1961) in a study of the social and psychological effects of disability in 41 children, ages seven to nineteen, hospitalized for some two years for the treatment of Legge-Perthes disease. It was assumed that self-perception of limitations in motor function would lower self-evaluation in the same way that the belief by the disabled that they are less worthy, less able or less attractive, may do. In the original form, a stimulus word or concept, *e.g.* Me, Cripple, Doctor, Mother, is placed at the top of a page and beneath it are listed a series of adjective pairs, *e.g.* hard-soft, strong-weak, large-small, separated by a 7-point scale. The adjective pairs have been found on factor analysis to fall into three main groups — evaluative, potency, and activity. The subject is instructed to choose a point on each scale line that they think best describes the word or concept at the top of the page.

In Downing's study the procedure was modified slightly by using a 5-point scale, 15 concepts, and 9 scales. Clifford has used the same procedure to study the differences between two subgroups of asthmatic children (1965a), focusing chiefly on the size of the differences between the concept of asthma and various self-concepts. In a second study, Clifford showed that children with cleft lip or palate placed themselves closer to the concepts of 'health' and 'cleft lip and palate' than to any of the other concepts listed. From his findings he concluded that these terms had become a part of the child's cognitive structure (1969).

Another group of techniques used to obtain indirect appraisals of self-evaluation are based upon level of aspiration. The general approach is to ask the child to predict how well he will do on some mental or physical task and then to compare this with actual performance. Harway (1962) used the Rotter board in a study of physically handicapped children and showed that the success predictions for this group of children differed from the findings of matched normal controls. The Rotter board is attractively designed like a miniature billiard table; a cue is used to try to place an object in a specified place.

In 1967, a novel method for assessing changes in self-concept during middle childhood was introduced by Long, Henderson, and Ziller. The test is based upon self-social personality theory which assumes that self-identity is derived from interpersonal orientations and experiences. Similarities and contrasts with others in the immediate social environment are considered necessary for a clear conception of the self. Five 'self-social constructs' are described to assess the schemata thought to be of importance during the period from about age 9 to 12 years. The important feature of this test is that it is essentially non-verbal — the child is given instructions orally and is able to respond by pointing to a circle, or pasting a circle on a page.

In their first report the authors described five such tasks to assess the following constructs — individuation, self-esteem, power, identification, and social dependency. In each instance, assertions are made about the interpretation of the manner in which the task is performed. For example, for individuation, a large circular area is presented containing a randomly placed array of small circles at the bottom of the page to represent himself; one of these is shaded and the others identical to the smaller circles above. The choice of the shaded, *i.e.* 'different' circle is interpreted as evidence of a higher degree of individuation. These assertions appear naive but in each case validation is offered which is surprisingly convincing. In their initial report the changes in relation to age and sex are described.

The interest of this procedure in relation to studies of adjustment lies chiefly in the construct claimed to assess self-esteem. It is based simply on the choice of one of eight circles in a row with positions to the left being assumed to represent a higher degree of self-esteem (Ziller *et al.,* 1969). Although the hypothesized relation with age was not found, subsequent studies led to a modification of the task — the circles being arranged in a row from top to bottom — and found to be related significantly to various cultural, ethnic and class characteristics. In a later study of adolescents, institutionalized because of behaviour problems, lower self-esteem was again found by comparison with normal controls. The procedure, and its interpretations, have been criticized by Carlson (1970) but numerous reports continue to appear describing the application of this unusual and attractively simple procedure. It has been employed in the Rochester studies of chronic illness and found to correlate with other measures of self-concept, but was not, however, as sensitive as Coopersmith's SEI, for example (Pless, 1975).

PROJECTIVE MEASURES

The third category of procedures are those designated as 'projective.' By this we mean that the respondent is presented with stimuli sufficiently ambiguous to permit him to 'project' thoughts, ideas and feelings, presumably from the unconscious. Most such measures are administered by a psychologist or psychiatrist as an adjunct to an unstructured, open-ended, probing interview. The responses so obtained always require interpretation, though in recent years there have been a number of attempts to standardize both administration and recording of responses in some of the more popular measures. Despite this, many psychometricians regard these measures with suspicion because they are so difficult to interpret, are of questionable validity, and generally of low reliability. Eysenck (1965b) has gone so far as to assert that there is no empirical data linking global projective test results with psychiatric diagnosis; that there is no consistent theory underlying these techniques; and that no evidence exists for their predictive power, either in relation to psychotherapy or in relation to success or failure in those activities in which personality factors are presumed to play a role. In spite of these criticisms, such procedures continue to be part of the standard repertoire of psychodiagnostics.

Table 5. **Measures to assess psychological adjustment of disabled children**

C. *PROJECTIVE MEASURES*
 1. *Figure Drawings*
   Draw-a-Person
     (Machover, 1949)
   Draw-a-Man
     (Goodenough, 1926)
   House-Tree-Person
     (Buck, 1948)
   Make-a-Picture Story Test
     (Hess, 1960)

II. *Sentence Completions*
       Incomplete Sentence Blank
           (Rotter, 1950)
  III. *Clinical Projectives*
       Rorschach Test
           (Rorschach, 1954)
       Structured Objective Rorschach
           (Stone, 1958)
       Thematic Apperception Test
           (Murray, 1943)
       Children's Apperception Test
           (Bellak and Bellak, 1955)
       Inkblot Technique
           (Holtzman, 1961)
       Picture Frustration Test
           (Rosenzweig, 1948)
       Picture Story Test
           (Symonds, 1964)
       Blacky Pictures
           (Taulbee, 1968)

Figure drawings

Of all the projective techniques, no single category is as frequently used as those involving simple drawings of people. The Draw-a-Person (Machover, 1951) is generally regarded as the most truly projective, although the Draw-a-Man, originally introduced in 1926 as a test of children's intelligence, has been restandardized by Harris (1961) for use in assessing personality. In the same broad category is Buck's House-Tree-Person (1948) projective technique for use with children five or older.

These drawing tests are each based on psychoanalytic assumptions; in physically disabled children one assumption is that the figure represents the child's perception of his body. There is also evidence, however, that drawings can be interpreted to indicate the child's anxiety (Fox *et al.*, 1958). The validity of these procedures remains equivocal and a major review by Roback (1968) of 18 years of research on the Draw-a-Person concluded that the case for or against their continued use remains essentially 'not proven'. This is so largely because the majority of validational studies have been poorly designed and better standardization is required.

There are numerous examples of the use of each of these

drawing tests in studies of children with chronic illnesses. Most often they are used in conjunction with other measures or combined with interviews, but occasionally the focus is exclusively to determine the body image through the drawing alone. Wysocki and Whitney (1965) describe one such attempt with 100 children, 50 of whom had orthopaedic disabilities. Fifteen aspects of the drawings were examined and six were found to be significant between the two groups (size, placement on page, shading, pressure, paper rotation and area of insult).

The DAP was also used in a wide variety of studies of adjustment in the chronically ill, e.g. Kahn et al.'s study of children with renal disease (1971); Reite et al.'s study of psychological function in osteogenesis imperfecta (1972); Schonfeld's study of body-image disturbances in adolescents with inappropriate sexual development (1964); and in Abercrombie and Tyson's study of children with cerebral palsy (1966). A more recent variant on the picture drawing theme has been introduced by Hess (1960) — the Make-a-Picture Story Test (MAPS). This has been used to study the adjustment of the deaf.

A second time-honoured category of projective measurement is the incomplete sentence procedure. This simple technique involves the use of neutral or ambiguous sentence stems which the child is asked to complete. For example, 'People think that I am . . .' or 'I think . . .' There are many such stems that have been designed by investigators for their own use. Although few have been standardized, one exception is the Rotter Incomplete Sentences Blank (1950) for use with children in grade nine and above. The sentence completion technique was also used by Cruickshank in his study of children with various physical disorders (1952) and in the Rochester studies. In the latter, the completions were scored according to the number of negative comments the child used, and the number of references to sickness or disability.

Clinical projective techniques

The more traditional projective techniques are used almost exclusively by clinical psychologists and psychiatrists. Two such measures have dominated the field since their inception — the Rorschach and the Thematic Apperception Test. In its original form, the Rorschach consists of 10 symmetrical, coloured inkblots. They are presented to the subject who is asked to describe what he sees. The responses are 'scored' in a number of ways, depending on the training of the examiner. In general, scoring takes account of the location, determinants and content of the responses. The intention is to interpret them in terms of the total configuration of ideas expressed, but in practice, there is little consistency in the manner in which the test is handled. One exception is the attempt by Stone (1958) to increase its objectivity. This measure, the Structured Objective Rorschach Test (SORT) was used by Goetzinger and his colleagues in a study of deaf adolescents (1966). Stone describes the SORT as 'a radical modification of traditional Rorschach Test.' Although it uses the same blots and basically the same scoring system and interpretative rationale, the SORT has no free responses and no inquiry. Instead it suggests responses and requires a fixed total number of them. In spite of the advantages claimed for this modification, most reports continue to refer to the traditional Rorschach in studies of the disabled (*e.g.* Olch, 1971b; Schonfeld, 1964).

The Thematic Apperception Test and the modification for children, the Children's Apperception Test (Bellak and Bellak, 1955) vie with the Rorschach in popularity. They require the subject to make up a story about each of a series of pictures showing people in various situations. It is assumed that the child will reveal his feelings, needs, motives and personality characteristics in the stories he creates. As with the Rorschach, attempts have been made to 'translate' essentially qualitative information into quantitative and, therefore, more objective data. Such a modification was employed by Mussen and Newman in their study of motivation and adjustment in physically handicapped children (1958). As a composite battery, Vigliano *et al.* (1964) coupled the CAT with the Holtzman Inkblot Technique and Symonds' Picture Story Test (1964) in their assessment of psychiatric sequelae of old burns in children.

The Inkblot Technique described by Holtzman *et al.* (1961)

has been used in a variety of ways to study handicapped children. One example is the development of two 'body boundary' indices — the Barrier Index and the Penetration Index, as used in the work of Myers and her colleagues in their study of girls with scoliosis (1970). Unlike the Rorschach, the Holtzman consists of two parallel forms; each comprises 45 inkblots, the responses to which are scored in terms of 22 variables. The procedure was also used in Koski's study of the coping processes in childhood diabetes (1969) along with Rosenzweig Picture Frustration Test.

The children's form of the Rosenzweig, described initially in 1948, consists of a booklet containing 24 cartoon-like drawings. Each drawing shows a person who is either frustrating a child in some fashion or pointing out improper behaviour on the part of the child. The remarks of the 'frustrator' are given and the subject is asked to supply what he feels would be an appropriate reply. The responses can be analyzed in a variety of ways.

Clinical interviews

Finally, although not properly a 'measure' in the usual sense of the term, mention must be made of psychiatric and psychologic interviews as a means of assessing adjustment. These interviews, particularly when they are standardized in some fashion, probably yield the maximum amount of information directly relevant to the question of adjustment. In the Isle of Wight survey, Rutter et al. (1970), studied all 10-to-12-year-old children with physical handicaps who had been screened by the parent and teacher checklists previously described. Psychiatrists interviewed each child, following a standardized procedure that had been shown to yield the same results when administered independently by two trained interviewers. Similarly, in their study of personality maturation in response to growth hormone treatment in hypopituitary dwarfs, Money and Pollitt (1966) obtained psychologic information through lengthy interviews, employing both 'direct and oblique questioning techniques.' They also made observations of the children's behaviour and 'way of relating to their peers, parents, and ward personnel during the period of hospitalization.'

Psychiatric evaluation of children with diabetes, based on a semi-structured interview, was used in conjunction with home interviews and a psychological test battery, to compare adjustment in these children with a group of matched healthy controls (Swift *et al.*, 1967). A similar procedure was followed by Sterky in his study of children with diabetes (1963).

Summary

This section has dealt with some of the methods employed to assess psychological adjustment in children with various chronic illnesses. Objective, subjective and projective procedures differ in the degree to which they examine overt behaviour as opposed to expressions of conscious or unconscious thoughts and feelings. In one respect, behaviour, whether observed by parents, teachers or an independent evaluator, may be regarded as the most pertinent form of such assessment. It could be argued, on that score, that so long as a child continues to perform well in everyday tasks, relates well to others and displays no overt manifestations of deviant behaviour, it matters little what he 'scores' on psychological tests or what fantasies he projects in response to various stimuli. On the other hand, since overtly disturbed behaviour represents already established or even advanced maladjustment, it is clearly important to identify deviance at an earlier stage if possible, both for therapeutic and investigative purposes. It is for this reason that subjective and projective measures, which are at once more subtle and refined, continue to attract their protagonists.

III

Long-term Adjustment to Chronic Disorder

Some relationship undoubtedly exists between behavioural patterns in childhood and adult functioning in a variety of spheres. The strength of this relationship, however, remains debatable. This section is, therefore, devoted to examining those consequences of chronic illness in childhood that occur during late adolescence or adulthood.

Two main mechanisms may be postulated — the first that psychological disturbance resulting from physical illness in childhood persists essentially unchanged; second, that even when there is no observable disturbance in the child, delayed developments may ultimately emerge that can still be traced to the original lesion. Of these two alternatives, the first is the more probable and the evidence for or against it stems most convincingly from studies of a longitudinal nature.

If there is such a link, the greater the probability that it leads to adult repercussions, the greater the interest likely to be shown by agencies responsible for adult care. While the problems of the handicapped child primarily affect his family, friends and teachers, they represent less of a burden in community terms than comparable adult handicap — such are the values of present-day society.

This pragmatic viewpoint is succinctly expressed by Merrill (1971), commenting on the prognosis for multiply-handicapped children as exemplified by his study of 32 cases. Sixty-two per cent of these had either died or were judged 'absolute failures.' Acknowledging the humane value of therapeutic support for such children and their parents, he nevertheless states '. . . to accept general support without more palatable success is a very limited goal . . . It seems more acceptable to establish as a goal the "graduation" of young adults . . . who are in a competitive position (so that they) thereby contribute to their own welfare . . . rather than represent a complete drain on (community) resources.'

In striking contrast to the abundance of studies describing problems of adjustment in childhood, however, there is paucity of evidence to help settle the important question of adult outcome. This lack of evidence reflects the enormous difficulty in mounting prospective or longitudinal studies; but it may also reflect a curious lack of interest on the part of paediatricians in the long-term results of their care. Whatever the case, the omission remains.

OPTIMAL ADJUSTMENT IN THE ADULT

As in childhood, the notion of psychological adjustment in adults is elusive and difficult to define. For most clinicians, the concept entails something other than 'superficial adaptation,' or 'passive acceptance' of the social reality. Perhaps, 'insight and mastery, a sense of acting on the internal and external environment, and Piagetian assimilation rather than mere accommodation,' better represent the qualities implicit in the clinician's use of the construct.

To define this notion more precisely, Siegelman, *et al.* (1970) studied 171 adults in their mid-30's followed from childhood as part of the Berkeley Guidance Study and the Oakland Growth Study. Each of the subjects was described by two or three psychologists using 90 California Q-set items. These were then compared with a hypothetical Q description of an 'optimally adjusted personality' previously obtained from nine experienced clinical psychologists. Thus, items such as 'warmth, capacity for close relationships, dependability, responsibility, insight, productivity, social perceptivity . . .,' etc. were taken to define optimal adjustment. Conversely, the most negative items included having 'a brittle ego-defense system; a small reserve of integration; disorganized and maladaptive when under stress; cheated and victimized by life; self-pitying; and lack of personal meaning'.

In this fashion a group of 'high' and 'low' optimally adjusted subjects were selected and differences examined in antecedent variables during childhood. The authors emphasize the salience of the mother's behaviour and adjustment; in particular her cognitive and coping skills. They conclude that the comparisons 'indicated unanimously healthy findings for the family relations of the high optimal adjustment subjects of both sexes.' In general, the families of origin of high optimal adjustment adults were 'more democratic, more open and direct, had greater sexual compatibility of parents, freer interchange of problems and feelings, greater agreement on values and important life areas, and greater orientation toward intangibles and the higher cultural values.' One interesting sex difference was also noted: although a precondition for good adjustment in both sexes seemed to be a competent and well integrated mother, poor adult adjustment required only a neurotic, anxious mother for boys, but two neurotic parents for girls. They also noted that the characteristics of the fathers of low 'optimal adjustment' females appeared to parallel those of the mothers of low optimal adjustment males.

This study is cited at some length because it represents a rarity in the field of personality research and forms a cornerstone for some of the reports that follow. Rarely does an opportunity exist to relate adult personality characteristics to *systematic* data obtained 25 years earlier on parent/child relationships and home characteristics. Although the design of the study has been criticized by Bronfenbrenner (1970) for its 'failure to illuminate adequately the differential influence of the two parents on the child of each sex,' it remains nevertheless a valuable contribution. Bronfenbrenner also takes issue with the researchers' apparent willingness 'to accept at face value the clinical evaluations on which so much of their data were based', calling into question their objective reality. He suggests that the measure of optimal adjustment used may well reflect a 'halo' effect based on the clinician's liking for the person in general.

These objections must be kept in mind as we examine further findings. On the other hand, no other study even attempts to tackle the notion of optimal adjustment globally. Instead, we are obliged to rely upon indirect or more limited indicators of specific components of adjustment. Such substitutes, it may be recalled, are necessary because examining childhood determinants of adult functioning calls for exceedingly difficult research. Mahrer (1969) stresses that 'although sporadic studies report occasional linkages, the major reviews of sound studies confirm that research evidence for any consistent relationships between childhood and adult personality is lacking.' As part of the solution to this shortcoming, Mahrer suggests that more attention be paid to multiple, interacting antecedent events rather than continuing to search in vain for single linkages. Similarly, he suggests that single events in childhood be examined in relation to a wider range of potential outcomes and this is essentially the strategy adopted in this section. Other suggestions offered by Mahrer include placing more emphasis on specific variables as opposed to global concepts, and examining more closely life processes that may act as mediators between childhood events and adult behaviour.

Several of these recommendations are reflected in the important report by Jones (1965) which is also based on part of the Oakland Growth Study. In this study an attempt is made to examine some of the psychological correlates of variations in somatic development, *i.e.* height, pubertal-height indices, strength, weakness, obesity, and onset of maturity. The major measures of psychological functioning are based on Gough's California Personality Inventory (CPI) administered to those still in the cohort at age 33 years (n=99). The findings are unusually conclusive: 'As a group, early maturing boys have assets that are valued in the peer culture — and these continue into adulthood.' 'Men who matured early describe themselves on the CPI as able to make a good impression, as poised, responsible, achieving in conformity with society's expectations, and as relatively free of neurotic symptoms.' In contrast, 'the boy whose pubescence came late is active and exploring with evidence of compensatory adaptations. In adulthood, he is insightful, independent, and impulsive.' These findings are consistent with much earlier reports (Barker *et al.*, 1953) suggesting that physique, somatotype, deviance in height and weight, each seemed to correlate to a small, but significant, extent with various adult behaviours. Many of these studies were carried out on prisoners or among college students, and although well executed, little note has been paid to their findings in recent years.

It is clear from other reports that some forms of adult

'functional impairment' can be predicted with reasonable accuracy from childhood indicators. In this sense, the term 'functional impairment' is used to describe disabilities of a physical, behavioural or academic nature. Most of this work, however, fails to examine the interaction between each of these childhood parameters and their potential adult outcomes. One reason for this is explained by Densen *et al.*, (1970) as follows:

They were concerned with the antecedents of rejections among young adults receiving examinations for the U.S. Selective Service System prior to military induction. In their studies they checked the school records and birth certificates of 3,511 subjects. They make the point, however, that 'rejection rates by cause cannot be used as measures of prevalence of medical or mental defects in the population examined, because of the way the examination procedure is carried out. Identification of a single cause for rejection of an examinee may terminate (the) process, leaving information on other possible causes incomplete.'

Nevertheless, the data from their study suggest that where problems do present in childhood they persist into early adulthood with sufficient regularity and severity to affect rates of military rejection. For example, 'more than 45% of examinees with heart defects in childhood, 42% of asthmatics or hay fever subjects, and 41% showing behavioral problems, were in fact rejected.'

Predictably, boys with two or more such problems had even higher rates of rejection. Such data might conceivably be attributed to the workings of the U.S. Selective Service System. They do, however, serve as a reminder that most of these childhood problems persist and hence the originally proposed mechanism is certainly tenable.

HOW LONG IS LONG-TERM?

The time scale adopted does, of course, vary in different studies. Broadly speaking, in this review, we have confined our interest to the age period 20 to 35 years because we felt that during this phase the potential consequences of maladjustment would be most crucial for subsequent career prospects, marriage and family building, vocational opportunities, etc. Beyond this age range the die is already cast. Nevertheless, we also include some studies on adolescent adjustment because we believe this period represents the final opportunity for preventive intervention by the paediatrician or his colleagues.

Were it to be shown, for example, that adolescents, say, with diabetes were much more disturbed psychosocially than their healthy peers, this would provide an additional impetus for therapeutic intervention at that stage on the assumption that otherwise there would be further deterioration with advancing maturational problems. On the other hand, because these teenage years are normally so full of flux, there is particular need for careful controls.

In the main, however, the studies reported here deal with illness that has begun early in childhood so that examination of adjustment during adolescence can be interpreted as an intermediate stage in the natural progression of the illness and its sequelae.

CONSEQUENCES DURING ADOLESCENCE

With certain reservations, to be elaborated elsewhere (p.171), we believe that the chronicity of the illness and the impact that it has on the child, his parents and his siblings is more significant than the specific character of the disorder, be it diabetes, cerebral palsy, haemophilia, etc. In other words, there are certain problems common to all chronic childhood illness over and above particular challenges posed by individual needs. Setting aside specificity of reaction for the present, therefore, we feel it worthwhile focusing upon some patterns of maladjustment during adolescence common to a variety of different chronic illnesses.

'Nuclear' psychiatric sequelae

Freeman (1970) epitomizes six years' clinical experience with handicapped adolescents, by claiming 'it is generally agreed that the incidence of psychiatric disorder is greater among the handicapped, and greater still during adolescence, but there is no good evidence that any one type of disturbance is universal or typical.' He cites Christy Brown's personal account of how it feels to be an adolescent with cerebral palsy. 'It was like living in chains . . . all the friendly ties that I had formed in my childhood were now broken by the rift that adolescence had wrought between myself and the boy I had played with as a child. It seemed that instead of coming to a better understanding of my handicap as I got older, I only became more troubled and bitter.'

Autobiographical accounts of this type are impressive and persuasive — up to a point. They cannot, however, be accepted as conclusive evidence that the group as a whole is more often disturbed than 'normal' adolescents. As pointed out by Shere and Kastenbaum (1954) for example, the non-affected sibling of the handicapped twin may be more frequently disturbed emotionally than the affected twin. Yet this too must not be interpreted uncritically since it draws attention to quite another aspect of the problem — the impact of the illness on other members of the patient's family and could be interpreted in this light.

Freeman lists a number of changes occurring in adolescence which could undermine previous adaptation to the handicap, in this case cerebral palsy. These factors include deterioration in the condition itself, the need to curtail certain fantasies about the possibility of cure, greater sensitivity to the attitudes of peers, the heightened importance of physical attractiveness during adolescence, problems associated with psychosexual maturation, schooling and school-leaving, but above all, the struggle for independence from parental control which in the case of the handicapped is inevitably heightened and complicated.

Despite these potentially powerful mechanisms, the actual evidence for higher incidence of psychiatric disturbance as such is surprisingly limited. In fact, in a number of studies of adolescents with diabetes, Collier (1969a) found no significant differences with matched healthy controls in respect to several personality traits as measured by the Interpersonal Check List (La Forge and Suczek, 1955). This study involved 125 matched pairs and employed sophisticated multivariate analysis of variance techniques to interpret the results. Essentially, only nine of the diabetics were found to have 'primary maladaptive behavior'. The author claims that his results support 'the contention that although adolescents with diabetes are subjected to the additional stress of their diabetes, the flexibility of their personality structure permits adaptation.'

In a subsequent publication, Collier (1969b) showed that adolescent diabetics are capable of academic achievement within the range of expected normality, and actually attained levels of achievement consonant with their abilities. (It is noteworthy, however, that in this study the majority of school personnel were not only aware of the child's illness but seemed to have a high degree of tolerance and understanding of it).

Suicide and suicidal intent

There is limited evidence to support the contention that suicide and suicidal intent may be more frequently encountered among adolescents with physical illness. In any case, it is claimed by Shrut (1964) that suicide is a major cause of death in adolescents and although girls make more 'attempts' than boys, male teenagers are more often successful. This apparent sex difference is related to the method of self-destruction selected. Among adolescents with medical illnesses, suicide threats are certainly frequent and often associated with the presence of pain. Weinberg (1970) describes a study of 13 patients, four boys and nine girls, all of whom had medical problems such as haemangioma, seizure disorder, diabetes, hypertension, etc. Each was studied systematically using a variety of measures including the TAT, and although no firm conclusions are drawn because of the small size of the sample, the author makes several important observations. He emphasizes, for example, the differing capacity to tolerate physical illness among boys compared to girls. Boys apparently conceive the illness as an obstacle to vocational or academic achievement. Whereas for the girls, the central theme seems to have been separation from critical figures.

Taking diabetes as an illustrative model, Stearns (1959) described three patients in their early twenties, all of whom had had diabetes since early childhood, to exemplify patterns of self-destructive behaviour. The problems he suggests, are not confined to overt suicidal attempts. Thus, frequent overdosages of insulin, deliberate omission of food, missing out on insulin shots or neglect of serious complications, might all be interpreted as subtly involving self-destructive trends.

Stearns cites corroborative evidence from other studies that while the incidence of overt suicide in diabetics of all ages was 0.3% prior to 1941, it rose to 0.5-0.7% during the period from 1922 — 1951. Without strictly comparable rates for the general population these figures mean little. Nevertheless, other investigators have noted the same phenomenon. In the suidical behaviour of three adolescent girls, for example, as described by Mason (1954), the presence of diabetes was noted as a background factor, while Rosen and Lidz (1949) have suggested that of 12 patients with repeated coma, 10 had 'actively or passively brought about acidosis in an attempt to escape difficult life situations.'

Educational achievement and performance

Another 'indirect' indication of maladjustment among chronically ill adolescents is their performance in school. Oddly enough, although frequent absence due to illness might be expected to impair scholastic performance, this has not been supported by objective findings. For example, in a major longitudinal study of a national sample, Douglas *et al.* (1968) have shown that examination performance at the time of school-leaving for the group as a whole was if anything rather better than in comparably placed pupils who are healthy, despite more frequent absence among the chronically ill patients.

This finding, however, may be qualified by severity of handicap. For example, studies of children with cerebral palsy show that at school-leaving age many with potentially normal intelligence had achieved far below that potential. Whether an indictment of the quality of teaching, or the educational milieu in special education classes or residential schools, or whether a consequence of the disease itself directly or indirectly, remains unclear. Indeed, the general debate over the alleged advantages of special education for the physically handicapped or 'delicate child' with normal intelligence is still unresolved (Pless, 1969; Pless, Rackham and Kellock, 1967; Anderson, 1974).

One facet of this issue is expressed admirably in the words of a young adult with cerebral palsy. 'I felt that too much emphasis, for me, was placed on the physical restorative activities, when I couldn't see that that would be of much help to me. I felt that more emphasis should be placed on what's being put into my head. I would be in arithmetic class and someone would come and say, "It's time for therapy" and they would pull you out of class.' (Richardson, 1972).

Support for this assertion is conflicting. Klapper and Birch (1966) describe a study of 155 children assessed initially between 1947 and 1948 and reviewed in 1962–63. At that time their ages ranged from 2 to 16 years. Eightynine of the original group were available for follow-up and of these, eleven had failed to complete elementary school while a further 22 had not completed high school. Taking into consideration the intellectual level of the group and their social backgrounds, the authors conclude that educational achievement is in line with what might be expected.

In her study of haemophiliacs, some of whom were adolescents, Olch (1971a) noted that their academic achievements were generally below ability levels and that these discrepancies increased with age. Although these children had frequent absences, the relationship between these and academic achievement was not a strong one. A similar conclusion was reached by Yule and Rutter (1970) in the Isle of Wight survey. Repeated short absences were noted among children with non-neurological chronic illness, and although this group performed less well on achievement tests standardized for intelligence, the association between these two findings was thought to be more probably mediated by other factors such as lack of motivation and loss of confidence.

In Katz' study of haemophiliacs (1970), 34% of the 1,055 young adults surveyed had not completed high school and 23% had received no further education. The similar conclusion is reached that academic achievement falls short of what might be expected for children of similar intelligence.

Vernon (1970) begins his review of the achievement of the deaf with the statement 'The most salient characteristics of low-achieving deaf persons is the overwhelming majority with normal potential.' He continues, 'There is no need for these persons to be low achievers. They represent a failure of education and other services and are testimony to a waste of human resources.' Based on a review of more than 50 studies, he claims it has been demonstrated conclusively that 'intelligence is distributed essentially the same in the deaf population as . . . among the non-deaf.' In stark contrast to this statement are the findings of four reports cited by him showing that educational achievement among deaf subjects is greatly below that of the hearing. For example, in the study by McClure (1966) of American deaf students over the age of 15, only 5% were achieving at tenth grade level or better and 60% were at Grade 5 level or below! Schein and Buschnaq (1962) estimate that only some 2% of deaf students attend college compared with some 10% of the hearing.

In a less detailed report, Thelander (1968) notes that only 35 children from a group of 184 cerebral palsy cases followed into adolescence from early childhood had IQ scores above 90. Their educational status as such is not described but the author implies that major learning problems exist even when the physical handicap is minimal and the IQs normal or above. Similar findings are reported by Rutter and Graham (1970) in the Isle of Wight survey and by Pollock and Stark (1969) in their analysis of the long-term results of 67 children with cerebral palsy. Only four were in universities or receiving higher levels of training in spite of the fact that 26 had IQ scores above 90. O'Reilly (1971) describes the status of 919 children with cerebral palsy of whom 38% were judged to have 'normal mentality.' Most of these were thought to be self-sufficient, and in his terms 'a large proportion . . . are able to complete regular school and to participate in normal activities.' However, no data is offered to support this assertion.

Among children with a variety of physical handicaps, the picture is even more confusing. Carlsen (1957) surveyed the status of 42 children who had attended a 'crippled children's school' from 1942 to 1955, using a postal questionnaire to which 31 responded. The age range of the group at the time of survey was between 14 and 33 years, the median IQ for those completing eighth grade was 95, and for those completing high school, 103. Only 21 of the group as a whole completed high school and of these, three proceeded with regular college training.

Children with cleft palate have been studied by Demb and Ruess (1967) to determine the frequency with which they 'drop out' of high school. The study was based on 64 children whose primary condition involved cleft lip or palate or both. Their educational patterns were compared with those of all siblings 17 years or older, and with rates for the general population of similar mean age (19.5 years). The most interesting finding is that by comparison with the national average rate of high school dropout (30%) the rate for children with clefts was 25% while that for their siblings was 42%! The drop-out rate was higher for boys with clefts (31%) than for girls (20%), but was identical for sibs of both sexes. There was no relation between the rate of drop-out and severity of the condition.

The other side of the coin is equally interesting. Forty-seven percent of the sibs were high school graduates and 3% college graduates, compared with only 37% of those with clefts. Moreover, the likelihood of remaining or dropping out of high school was similar within families. This suggests that the determining factor is the interaction between family characteristics and the presence of the condition, rather than the condition *per se*.

Demb and Ruess conclude by restating a central theme of this section. 'During the past 20 years there has been a paucity of systematic studies . . . regarding the psychosocial functioning of cleft palate persons beyond the adolescent stage. Virtually all workers in this field would probably agree that the goal of any, and all, habilitative procedures is to maximize the child's potential and minimize the effects of the congenital disability in order to obtain optimum psychosocial functioning at maturity. Yet, there are no extant data to show whether this goal is being attained . . . When, and if, future studies are completed, it may be found that some of the current practices, assumptions, and emphases of treatment may not always enhance or maximize the potential of many cleft palate children for coping with the developmental tasks of adulthood.'

Some light may be thrown upon these apparent discrepancies through a number of reports not primarily related to ill children. Simmons, *et al.* (1973) in a major cross-sectional study of nearly 2,000 urban children, show that early adolescence, *i.e.* ages 12-13 years, is a period of much greater self-consciousness, greater instability of self-image, lower self-esteem and less favourable view of the opinions held of themselves by 'significant others.' Is it not likely, therefore, that the child with a chronic illness is especially vulnerable at this time and, therefore, even less able to cope with the demands imposed by a new, secondary school setting?

Although perhaps tangential to the issue, the work of Dalton (1968) might help to explain some of the effects of illness on school performance. A study of examination results of girls shows that significantly lower average marks are obtained during the premenstruum. The effect was even greater among those girls with lengthy menstrual periods or long menstrual cycles. If such a normal variation in physiology can have so significant an effect on academic performance, is it not remarkable that the overlay of chronic illness seems to have such minimal and inconsistent effects in the same area of performance?

Finally, a brief look at the reverse side of the picture — the effect of the disability on the perception and judgment of the evaluator. An important study by Canning and Mayer (1966) raises the possibility that obesity may influence the judgment of the interviewer and thereby affect the adolescent candidate's chance of a college place. In this study of 1,165 students in high school graduating classes, although academic criteria and application rates for obese and non-obese students were equivalent, there were significantly fewer obese students accepted into college. The differences were particularly marked for female students. Twenty-three per cent of the high school female population were obese compared with 11.2% of the college students, whereas 18% of high school boys were obese compared with 13.7% of college boys.

Because grades, application rates, and social classes were comparable between obese and non-obese students, the authors claim a 'Strong possibility . . . that a form of unconscious prejudice toward obese adolescents is exercised by high school teachers in writing recommendations, or by college interviewers, or both.' The observation is reported to emphasize the complexity of factors involved in examining this single indicator of successful adjustment during adolescence.

CONSEQUENCES DURING ADULTHOOD
Criminality and other forms of deviance
Relatively little interest was shown in the relationship between abnormalities of physique and various deviant behaviours, until reports began to appear in the mid-60's emphasizing the frequency of behaviour problems among adults with Klinefelter's syndrome (XYY chromosome disorder) (Hook, 1973). Since this condition is inherited genetically, it must be included among the chronic disorders of childhood. Is such behaviour a direct manifestation of the chromosomal disorder (and hence, biologically determined) or is it mediated through the psychosocial consequences of the unusual deviation in physique which the abnormality produces? Some answers are provided by Nielson and Tsuboi (1970) in their study. All 771 male patients in a psychiatric hospital were examined and their stature, criminal records, and history of alchohol or drug abuse noted. One of the principal findings was that nearly 25% of patients with 'character disorders' equalled or exceeded a stature of 181 cm. Clear evidence of criminal behaviour was found disproportionately among this group of tall patients, particularly in the younger age range. A link between such deviant behaviour and tall stature, in association with the XYY syndrome, was also shown in this study and in earlier ones. Again the criminal conduct is especially prevalent among the 10-19-year-old patients, either those with XYY syndrome or those with tall stature alone.

The only other medical condition in childhood frequently linked to deviant behaviour in later life is epilepsy. Apart from well-established instances in which the epilepsy is secondary to definite cerebral damage with consequent retardation, this link is largely a reflection of folklore and superstition. Gunn and Fenton (1971) examined all epileptic patients who were inmates of a large prison hospital in Britain, as well as reporting on the findings from a national survey of epileptic prisoners. The first point of note is that the prevalence of epilepsy among male prisoners is between seven and eight per 1,000. Although this accords closely with rates among children, it is significantly higher than the anticipated rate in the general adult male population. No particular type of crime or pattern of criminal behaviour is found to be associated with epilepsy which raises the question as to whether 'automatism' might account for the higher frequency of epilepsy among prisoners. From their study, Gunn and Fenton were able to conclude that 'automatic behaviour' is a rare explanation for the crimes of epileptic patients. Although they do not say so themselves, it is interesting to speculate that criminal behaviour among epileptics may be another genuine example of maladjustment. As such it could reflect, albeit indirectly, the psychosocial consequences of a chronic illness which often begins in childhood. Might it not be equally rewarding to look for evidence of increased frequency of other long-term illnesses of childhood among populations of criminals, drug addicts, alcoholics, etc.?

Marital and sexual adjustment

Another oblique indication of maladjustment, given adequate controls, might be the frequency of prolonged bachelorhood or spinsterhood. These assume that marriage is a 'normal' outcome of development to maturity, but as such, open to question. For large groups, however, the observation that the marriage rate is significantly less among the handicapped may, nonetheless, be interpreted as further evidence for their failure to adjust normally. This is not to imply that this failure is theirs alone; in this area more perhaps than any other, the prejudicial attitudes of society undoubtedly play some role.

There is certainly evidence that marriage rates are lower among those who have had chronic illnesses since childhood. Brieland (1967) found for example, that only 24% of 67 students with various orthopaedic handicaps had married — an even higher rate than the less than 20% reported in several other comparable studies of children with similar disabilities. Bronks and Blackburn (1968) in their study of haemophiliacs, found that of 85 patients of marriageable age, 49% were, or had been married. Lambert *et al.*, in a follow-up study of juvenile amputees (1969) found a similar proportion; 49% were married at the time of their study. Virtually the same results emerged in Spencer's study (1968) of 26 haemophiliacs whose mean age at the time was 30: 42% were, or had been married. However, a high proportion of these were subsequently separated or divorced, or were having marital or sexual problems. In his very large scale study of more than 1,000 haemophiliacs, Katz (1963) found that 46% had married and, at the time of the study, only 2.2% were divorced or separated. The data from Carlsen's study, however, suggest a much lower rate of marriage — 12%, and, although figures are not given, Vernon (1969b) cites findings from Rainer's study of the deaf (1963) to indicate 'a slightly higher percentage of unmarried persons among the deaf' (which he attributes, in part, to the somewhat high ratio of men to women among the deaf). He also notes that most deaf persons marry other deaf persons and suggests that this represents a healthy adjustment to deafness.

These figures on rates of marriage are difficult to interpret in the absence of comparable rates for non-disabled adults of similar age and social background. It is perhaps significant that some relation seems to exist with the nature and severity of the disability and also with the date of the study. In general, disabilities affecting the nervous system and those with major locomotor components seem to affect marriage rates more adversely than do those with relatively milder, less overt handicaps; and, further, the rates seem uniformly higher in the more recent studies. The opportunity for marriage is probably a better indicator of the attitudes and prejudices of the non-disabled than a reflection of 'adjustment' in the disabled.

Psychological symptoms and psychological test results
Properly executed, studies comparing the frequency of abnormal psychological symptoms or test results among adults whose disabilities began during childhood with those of comparable healthy persons, provide a fairly direct indication of degree of maladjustment experienced by the disabled.

However, the studies in this area are as uneven as in most other spheres. Much depends on the tests used and how appropriate their application to special groups.

In an unpublished study, for example, Muthard (1963) compared the MMPI profiles of a group of 76 college students with cerebral palsy of varying severity with available norms for persons of the same age and sex. The group studied was a stratified random sample of subjects with this disorder and the tests were carefully administered. The author was aware of the need for cautious interpretation based upon previous studies which had highlighted too familiar pitfalls. Muthard's results, however, suggest that 'male cerebral palsied college students react to the demands of college with a greater amount of worry, feelings of worthlessness, seclusiveness, and feelings of inferiority than their female counterparts. Both men and women showed mean response patterns which were deviant when compared to norms for college men and women. The results suggest that they are more emotionally disturbed and in need of pyschological help than their non-impaired peers.' This conclusion is based on the clinical keys of the MMPI, and the Mt scale intended for use specifically with college students. Also used as an index of maladjustment is the number of scales with T scores exceeding 70 — 46% of the CP men and 29% of the women had two or more scaled in this range. The scores are interpreted by Muthard (1965) as suggesting that the disabled chiefly have problems of social group acceptance — a not unexpected finding. It is also of interest, however, to note no significant relationship with the degree of impairment based on self-ratings of severity.

These findings may be contrasted with the work of Stone *et al.* (1966) who obtained MMPI data from adolescents with a variety of organic disorders and found profiles almost identical to the norms for children of similar age. The MMPI was also used by Stehbens and MacQueen (1973) in a follow-up survey of children with proven rheumatic (Sydenham's) chorea. Sixty-five children (19 boys and 46 girls) were found who had experienced this illness on average, 10 years earlier. These were matched by sex and age with children who had no such illness. Only one significant difference was found between the two groups — the K (Correction Scale), denoting a circumspect, social desirability set personality attribute, was higher among females with chorea. Both this study and that of Sacks et al. (1962) are of interest in comparison with the more extensive work of Wertheimer (1963) (p.78) in which rates of psychiatric treatment for patients with this disorder were found to be elevated.

In their appraisal of maladjustment in haemophiliacs, Bruhn et al. (1970) employed three psychological tests — Rotter's IE scale (a measure of internal vs. external control); the Maudsley Personality Inventory, providing measures of neuroticism and extraversion; and the Personal Adjustment Sub-scale of the Adjective Check List of Gough and Heilbrun. (A test of Family Adjustment was also included but not as a measure of adjustment.) The tests were shown to be independent of each other and hence are presumed to assess different aspects of psychological adjustment.

The results showed more internal control and neuroticism for the group as a whole; however, more significant deviations were found for the 'marginally severe' than for either the mildly or severely disabled among the group studied. (The marginal group was less extraverted than the other groups and more externally controlled.) These findings are consistent with the theories of the somatopsychologists who postulate that the conflict imposed in marginal situations is particularly important in the maladjustment that follows physical handicap in some instances. [Similar findings have been reported for children with arthritis by McAnarney et al. (1974) and by Cowen et al. (1961) for adolescents with visual disorders.]

Although only about one-half of the patients studied had the onset of their illness before the age of 15, a study by Murawski et al. (1970) of the personality patterns in patients with diabetes mellitus, is also of interest in this regard. One hundred and twelve patients with diabetes of longer than 25 years duration were studied. Sixty-seven had been awarded a Medal in recognition of the absence of peripheral vascular, renal or retinal vascular complications. The principal purpose of the study was to compare the personality of those who had presumably succeeded in maintaining good control of their disease (thereby avoiding sequelae) with those who failed to do so. The MMPI was again the measure chosen for this purpose. The results are presented separately for male and female medallists and non-medallists.

For all four groups the scores were within 2 standard deviations of the mean, but were high (around or above 1 SD) for Depression and Hysteria and low on the scale for Social Introversion. Only one scale, the hypochondriasis scale, differentiated between medal and non-medal patients, with non-medal patients of both sexes having higher scores.

The authors interpret their results in the light of Treuting's review (1962) which concluded that 'although emotional states affect the course of the illness, the illness itself produces some of the observed emotional problems.' The depression score is probably a consequence of the disease rather than in any sense aetiologic. The group as a whole are characterized by seeking out and enjoying the company of others and perhaps having a greater need for contact with others. They also note that 'feelings of pessimism, hopelessness, and depression were quite strong' and found it difficult to sort out the significance of the hypochondriasis findings in relation to cause or effect. The authors conclude that the general trends found 'might be expected with any chronic disease which affects the total fabric of a person's life and pleasures.' The differing significance of this illness for men and women is often ignored in studies of this kind. The findings may be viewed as providing some indication of the psychological price paid in order to achieve good symptomatic control. Those who stress the importance of 'tight' control in order to prevent organic complications must take the possibility into account that to achieve such control many psychological stresses are imposed on the child and his family.

The issue of the effects of treatment on psychological outcome during adulthood has also been considered by Feinstein and his colleagues (1962) in relation to rheumatic heart disease. The focus in this study of 216 patients followed for an average of 21 years after an attack of rheumatic fever, was on the restrictions of activity imposed by the physician in an effort to protect the heart. It was found that the objective cardiac status was essentially the same among those whose activities were restricted as among those permitted to engage in normal activities. Of interest in the context of psychological adjustment, however, are the results regarding psychosocial effects based on information obtained during an interview with the patients. The information included changes in schooling or scholastic ambitions, changes in occupational conditions or plans, alteration in marital plans, number of children, etc. It was found that adverse psychosocial effects were much more frequent among those children who had had restrictions imposed on their activities, whether or not cardiac involvement was present. Although recommendations are made for the management of patients depending on the presence or absence of cardiac enlargement, the general conclusion is reached 'that most restrictions are of dubious value' and that 'no useful purpose is served by many of the scholastic, athletic, vocational, and other physical restrictions that are often imposed upon the asymptomatic post-rheumatic fever patient.' These restrictions, they add, 'may create unpleasant psychosocial effects that negate any of the anticipated medical advantages.'

Psychiatric symptoms and rates of referral

The most direct indication of psychological maladjustment is the need for psychiatric treatment. Because not all those who need such treatment seek it or are able to receive it, the presence of symptoms judged by psychiatrists to be significant is as important as the actual fact of therapy having been provided. When these symptoms occur during adult life following a chronic illness that was present during childhood it may be assumed that a causative relationship exists (with the reservations already discussed). In the case of certain illnesses, particularly those involving the nervous system, the association may be interpreted as an expression of organic brain disorder.

The important follow-up study by Wertheimer (1963) compared the frequency of psychiatric diagnoses, both 'organic' and 'functional' among young adults who, as children had rheumatic chorea and other chronic illnesses. Wertheimer had theorized that because rheumatic chorea involves the nervous system, and is occasionally manifested by emotional disturbances, and because studies of schizophrenia had shown an association with theumatic fever (RF), it was possible that subsequently diagnosed 'functional' mental disorders may in fact represent repeated attacks of atypical chorea or the sequelae of these. She predicted, therefore, that children with rheumatic fever during puberty would display more psychiatric difficulties subsequently when compared with children who had RF at other ages, or children with other chronic diseases who had been selected as controls.

The design of the study was retrospective: males over the age of 24 years, who had a hospital record of this and other chronic diseases, were selected and the records of mental institutions throughout the state were searched for indications that they had received treatment. A sample of 595 cases from New York State and 2,092 cases from Colorado were used, the former containing names of children with RF and chorea and their siblings, the latter, in addition, the names of children with diabetes, tuberculosis, orthopaedic conditions and a random sample of hospital admissions and school children. Both samples included all available cases of the disorder in question from each institution studied who were born within a specified time period, thus insuring that they were under the age of 18 at the time of hospitalization. Since all cases were aged 24 or older at the time of the study, only psychiatric contacts at this age or earlier were studied.

The author carefully considers sources or error (death, migration, clerical errors, etc.) including possible bias on the part of the investigator. The most important consideration is the fact of it being highly unlikely that all or even most cases of psychiatric disorder, especially those from the lower social classes, will have received treatment and further, that not all treatment is provided by state institutions. Nevertheless, these errors are probably distributed evenly among each of the subgroups and efforts have been made to take them into account in interpreting the results.

These results show that both those with rheumatic chorea, as postulated, and those with other chronic disorders, have higher rates of psychiatric disorder than do the healthy controls or siblings. The average rate of 'functional' psychiatric disorder among controls between the ages 12 to 24 years is 2.3%. That figure is nearly doubled for children with non-rheumatic disorders (4.0%), being highest for those with congenital disorders (5.7%) and lowest for the post-polio cases (2.9%). The rate for siblings of children with rheumatic disease in the New York sample was 3.0% compared with 4.9% for those with RF alone, and 6.6% for those with chorea. In the Colorado study the rate for children with RF alone was 6.3% and for those with chorea was 9.4%. (Interestingly, the siblings of the rheumatics had a rate of 7.4% — more than three times the figure for the healthy controls and nearly twice that for those with non-rheumatic chronic disorders.) The results pertaining to the frequency of 'organic' psychiatric disorders, *e.g.* mental defectives, seizures, or those with a diagnosis of 'rheumatic brain disease', and those pertaining to psychiatric illness under the age of 12 are not discussed here because they cannot be viewed as long-term psychological consequences of chronic illness in childhood.

Wertheimer interprets her findings, especially in the light of further analysis of age-specific psychiatric rates, as support for her thesis that 'pubertal rheumatic disease leads to organic mental disorders which, because of lack of clear and typical organic symptomatology, are often diagnosed as "functional". The data are impressive but the conclusion does not necessarily follow. As the author herself points out, the high rates found among pubertal rheumatics may well reflect the psychological trauma of such an illness during this period. Examined in this light, with equal attention focused on children with other chronic diseases, it is significant that both the frequency of psychiatric treatment and the diagnoses made, differ when the various sub-groups are compared with the 'disease free' controls. Single contacts were from 3 to 8 times more frequent among all the chronically ill compared with the controls, whereas more intensive contact was only increased significantly for those with RF or 'potential RF'. Psychoneurotic disorders were nearly three times as frequent among those with non-rheumatic chronic disorders (1.3% vs. 0.5% for the controls) and was also greater among those with chorea and the 'potential RF' cases, whereas increased rates of antisocial behaviour diagnosis were found for those with RF.

These findings are presented in detail because they derive from the most extensive follow-up study to date. In smaller studies of a similar retrospective nature, a high frequency of psychiatric consultations has been noted for young adults with juvenile rheumatoid arthritis and those with diabetes (Pless, 1966). Spencer's study of 26 patients with haemophilia (1968) found that 23% had 'frank psychiatric symptoms' including alcoholism, depression, antisocial behaviour, psychosis and drug addiction. In the absence of suitable controls, however, it is difficult to know what to make of this finding. The questionnaire by Bronks and Blackburn (1968) of 135 patients with haemophilia showing only 6 patients (4.5%) willing to state that they had consulted a psychiatrist, is more likely to reflect limitation in the method used than to be a true statement of the frequency of mental illness among this group of patients. Rainer's extensive survey of deaf persons included some data about the frequency of psychosis to show that mental illness of this severity does not have an excessively high prevalence (1963). With respect to lesser mental disturbances, however, there was some evidence for higher prevalence of problems relating to impulse control and lack of insight (Vernon, 1969a). Comparably extensive surveys of children with chronic illness followed into adulthood include that of Katz (1963) who has studied more than 1,000 adults with haemophilia, and Pless *et al.* (1975) who have studied children with a variety of chronic physical disorders as part of a national cohort born in 1946. In the haemophilia study, little mention is made of psychiatric disorder as such. Those who have never been employed are regarded as 'socio-psychologically disabled' and it is assumed that their 'self-concept is that of a chronically handicapped person and, therefore, a social deviant.' In the study by Pless *et al.*, a higher proportion of the chronically ill had received psychiatric attention by the age of 26 years compared with the remaining members of the cohort. But the differences are only significant for particular sub-groups characterized by particular types of disability combined with greater degrees of severity.

Vocational achievements, employment and productivity
At the beginning of this section, we suggested that the most important aspect of maladjustment in adult life might well be the extent to which it interferes with the patient's ability to be self-sufficient. As in the case of marriage, however, as an

index of maladjustment, so with employment problems experienced by the chronically ill — they cannot be regarded as a direct manifestation of psychosocial inadequacy. The attitudes of employers are of obvious importance, these, in turn being affected by the social climate of the community and the economics of the period. Thus, to base 'success' in medical management upon the prospect of achieving stable, productive employment by the handicapped is to impose unrealistic standards for their care. This is not to decry, however, the overriding importance of self-sufficiency stemming from such an achievement.

In an unusual follow-up study of 27 young adults with congenital heart disease aged between 19 and 30 years (mean age 23 years), Goldberg and Satow (1972) showed vocational plans to be a good predictor of actual achievement. Those with realistic plans, *i.e.* in keeping with previous education and aimed at long-range goals, were motivated to 'obtain, maintain or redirect their employment to conform with . . . capabilities as . . . affected by their cardiac status.' Based on a Scale of Vocational Adjustment questionnaire administered as a semi-structured interview, the authors argue that patients with 'vocational maturity' were influenced more by intrinsic desires and interest and less by the opinions of others. Good vocational planning was found more often where interest had not been restricted unduly on account of illness, or to be associated with higher levels of education. None of these findings is particularly surprising nor in any sense conclusive; but, unlike some other studies, while level of disability did not significantly correlate with vocational measures as such, they did relate to intermediate factors such as restriction in interests, pessimism in outlook, etc.

More clear-cut conclusions are reached by Vernon (1969b) in his extensive review of the sequelae of adult deafness. 'Despite having the same intelligence as hearing people,' he states, 'deaf people frequently enter into manual labour of varying skill levels because they have no opportunity to engage in appropriate higher level employment.' Based on extensive national studies, Vernon notes that approximately 80% of the deaf are in some form of manual labour, in contrast to some 50% of the general population. At the other end of the employment spectrum, only 17% of the deaf do white-collar work compared with 46% of the general population. This striking evidence of the consequences of one disabling chronic disorder, commonly beginning in childhood, but with vocational implications, is undoubtedly due to one main factor — the failure of special educational programmes these children almost invariably receive. To a lesser degree, but nonetheless important, is the psychological damage inflicted on the deaf child's developing personality and self-concept, coupled with society's prejudices toward the deaf. Discussing the significance of these findings, Vernon (1970) claims that 'applying for positions is an Achilles heel to most deaf persons, regardless of their vocational or professional competence. Because of their frequent speech problems, even among those . . . adept at lip reading, the job interview . . . (can be) so embarrassing and distressing that deaf persons often take inferior positions, or else remain . . . in jobs far beneath their capabilities due simply to the trauma . . . (of) applying for a job.'

Other studies point to equally disappointing employment prospects even for groups with more 'socially acceptable' handicapping disorders. For example, both the report by Brieland (1967) and that of Carlsen (1957) describing a variety of orthopaedic or mixed physical handicaps in young adults suggest that employment rates are well below their probable intellectual abilities. Brieland reports only 46% of the group of 41 'graduates' from a special residential school programme as being employed at the time of the study; the rate for women being significantly higher than for men (69% vs. 37%). This report demonstrated a direct relation to severity of disability, although adequacy and availability of transportation are also mentioned. Carlsen's study endorsed these findings. She reports that 67% of graduates from the special school surveyed who only had an eighth grade education were unemployed, whereas for those completing college, only 28% were unemployed. Both studies are of small, probably unrepresentative samples; they may thereby present a bleaker picture than exists among the disabled population as a whole. They do suggest, however, that those who find their way into residential school programmes for whatever reason, face a grim future in the working world.

The importance of severity of disability as a determinant should not be underestimated. Most studies on the fate of children with cerebral palsy reveal that ultimate employment prospects are extremely poor, and that when employment is secured it is frequently at a much lower level than that of non-disabled persons of equal intelligence. Several British studies (Pollock and Stark, 1969; Ingram *et al.* 1964) plus the USA study by Klapper and Birch (1966) support this general observation. The purpose of Pollock's study was to determine the extent to which a special residential school programme (Westerlea in Scotland) had succeded in fitting these children to take their place in society. Of the 75 former pupils followed up, 48 were beyond school age, 18 of them having IQ's above 90. Only 9 of this group were in open employment, 1 was at University and 5 were in either 'token' or 'sheltered' employment or regarded as unemployable. Similarly, in their extensive Scottish survey, Ingram *et al.* found that only 21% of the 200 patients surveyed were in 'open employment', while 44% were unemployed. It is important to note that the majority of those in open employment had only mild to moderately severe disabilities. In contrast, those previously employed but latterly not working, although no more seriously disabled, were of somewhat lower intelligence on the average (26 of the 43 in open employment had IQ scores of 90 or above). The majority of those who were working did not consider themselves as handicapped. Significantly, although the majority of this group had parents whose attitudes toward their child's handicap was judged to be 'realistic', many were described as 'denying', or 'unrealistic', whereas only two were labelled 'over-protective.' Hence, although this study was not intended to highlight the importance of self-attitude and parental attitude in influencing prospects for ultimate employment, the results in fact indicate that 'denial' can be of positive value in promoting more effective self-acceptance (given certain safeguards).

The survey by Klapper and Birch included 89 young adults with cerebral palsy who were part of a group of 155 children studied originally in 1948. Only 15 of the 80 who were over the age of 18 years were in competitive employment, and of these only 3 were truly financially independent. More than one-half were unemployed and over 60% were completely dependent on their families financially. These findings must be examined in the context that more than 50% had completed high school and 9 had received college or grade school education beyond the high school level. The authors note that employment level was largely related to self-care status and hence to the severity of disablement. As to the importance of schooling, it is noted that 'there was no instance of skilled employment in any individual whose schooling had not gone as far as high school graduation . . . with higher education the cerebral palsied young adult would be more likely to find some kind of employment, but even with such educational advantages the likelihood of obtaining skilled employment was remote.'

The importance of higher education is emphasized by Reed and Cantoni (1966) in their study of handicapped college graduates. Of the 53 respondents in the study, representing a diverse set of disabilities, 52 were working at the time of the study, chiefly in the field for which they were prepared. Their major occupations were in education, rehabilitation counselling or social work, but some were in such highly specialized fields as engineering and computer programming. Almost as impressive are the results reported by Lambert *et al*, (1969) in their follow-up of children who had an amputated limb. Of the 150 patients studied, 112 were gainfully employed, 28 were students and only 2 were not working.

Among groups with relatively less severe disabilities, such as haemophiliacs, vocational achievements tend to be more useful as an indirect indicator of adjustment. Thus, the survey by Katz of more than 1,000 adult haemophiliacs (1963) showed that some 53% were employed. More noteworthy, perhaps is the fact that fully 20% were unemployed or had never been employed despite the relatively mild degree of handicap produced by this disorder. That this reflects difficulties in adjustment is further evidenced by the finding that of those employed, only 24% held 'white-collar' jobs, and in general 'no clear relationship was found between severity of illness and occupation'. In their study of 135 adult haemophiliac patients in the UK, Bronks and Blackburn (1968) noted that 65% of the clinically severe group were in employment (more than half had been at work for over 60% of the preceding 5 years); patients with less severe illness apparently had an even better work record. The authors comment that the findings 'bear witness to the determination of patients to succeed in the face of prolonged adversity and to the efforts of many workers in the treatment and rehabilitation fields'.

Summary

The consequences of a childhood chronic disorder that are manifest during adult life vary enormously. There are undoubtedly many instances where even children with severely disabling disorders lead a functionally and psychologically 'normal' adult life. But there are many more, it would seem, whose failure to adapt or cope successfully during childhood is carried over into later life. In such cases the ultimate results may be extremely grave, since psychosocial handicap in adult life, combined with some degree of physical disability, frequently appears to result in prolonged, forced dependence on family and ultimately on society. The costs of this degree of dependency are incalculable and further investigations are certainly warranted to establish more clearly the antecedents of such an outcome and, more important, to establish appropriate means of intervention that may prevent these undesirable long-term effects of childhood illness.

IV

Short-Term Adjustment to Chronic Disorder

Evidence does exist that some children with chronic illnesses are more vulnerable to psychosocial disturbance than their healthy peers, but it is scattered and of variable quality, and much of it is anecdotal, largely based on clinical experience. There is, however, a growing number of well-designed scientific studies which support the same conclusion.

The first part of this section focuses upon heterogeneous groups of the chronically sick with special emphasis on scholastic performance as an indirect index of maladjustment. The second part deals with specific disorders broadly categorized by types of lesion or forms of disability with differing psychological significance. These include (a) disorders involving the central nervous system; (b) disorders of the special senses — speech, hearing and vision; (c) cosmetic disorders; (d) locomotor problems and (e) organ system or systemic illnesses, *e.g.* diabetes, haemophilia, heart disease, asthma. In the third part, common threads are traced between these various groups, to help in formulating therapeutic guidelines.

Few, if any, major chronic childhood disabilities are associated with *specific* emotional or social patterns of disturbance. At any rate, none of the recent detailed surveys (Rutter, *et al.*, 1970; Dinnage, 1970, 1972; Pilling, 1973) uncover evidence to this effect. These studies do, however, testify to the emotional impact a chronic illness may have both on the child and on his family.

In contrast to the group studies, however, studies of individual children show that *any* physical disability may have a profound effect on behaviour. Several authors also make the point that the effect of illness on behaviour is not invariably adverse. When, for example, the disability has 'protective and rewarding consequences' the result may be good social and emotional adjustment. This must be kept in mind when examining data from group studies since the results from such aggregate data, may, in effect cancel out statistically. Consequently, if some children's behaviour is worsened and others is improved, the net effect may be to show little change whatsoever.

But why do some children appear to adjust positively to the stress of chronic illness while others fail to do so? We believe that all these children are at greater risk for maladjustment, yet the determinants of individual outcome are extremely complex and difficult to predict. Not all are equally at risk, so that our major task is to identify those who are most vulnerable at the earliest possible time. Our ability to do so and thereby intervene successfully, may prove, in the long run, the most important aspect of the care provided.

'A child born with a congenital defect has to face not only (its) crippling anatomical and physiological effects but also the emotional reaction of his family and of society — a reaction which may be even more crippling to his total emotional and physical growth than the physical defect itself.' (Easson, 1966). Further, Korsch (1958) has observed that 'The psychologic implications of chronic illness have been more extensively discussed in the literature than has acute illness, for readily understandable reasons, since limitations in specific organic therapy lead to more concern with other therapeutic approaches. Moreover, the long-term relation of physician, patient, and family in cases of chronic illness makes for increasing awareness of the psychologic needs of patient and family and of the paediatrician's psychotherapeutic role. Finally, the paediatrician's traditional interest in growth and development motivates him to study the effects of illness on development.'

A major physical illness for most children represents a psychological crisis and, as Caplan has suggested, crises provide opportunities for maturation if they are responded to appropriately. The excellent autobiographies by disabled persons (as listed for example by Pless and Satterwhite, 1971),testify not only to triumph in the face of adversity, but to positive accomplishments which may never have taken place were it not for the crisis so engendered. Similarly, there are families who, far from being devastated by the birth of a defective child, describe ways in which the event in retrospect proved to be a 'blessing in disguise.' The frequency of this phenomenon has never been quantified to our knowledge; but the likelihood remains that often it is an elaborate rationalization to help the family cope with the trauma of the event. Nevertheless, the fact is that handicapping illness does not invariably result in maladjustment. On the contrary, it may, on occasion, provide the stimulus for developing new skills, new talents or the growth of personality.

GENERAL STUDIES OF ADJUSTMENT

In his discussion of the socio-psychological consequences of handicapping, Richardson (1963) focuses on the effects of chronic disability upon a person's social development and capacity for human relations. Two questions are raised: first, whether handicapping has a 'blunting' or a 'sensitizing' effect; and second, whether specialized skills need to be developed by the handicapped to manage social relationships with the non-handicapped. With respect to the first, Richardson cites empirical studies to illustrate how handicaps (such as cerebral palsy) restrict the child's opportunity for exploration, spontaneous behaviour and social experience. The net effect is in the direction of 'blunting', *i.e.* impoverishing the child's resources for dealing with others. With respect to special interpersonal skills, Davis (1961) has described various stages in the development of a personal relationship with the non-handicapped. Each is accompanied by definite strategies and associated techniques to facilitate coping in face-to-face encounters. Although these examples provide convincing evidence from among handicapped adults, there is little to suggest whether the same kind of skills are used by children, and if so, the age at which they are learned.

The significance of the stage of development is also stressed by Maddison and Raphael (1971). They draw upon the work of others (*e.g.* Garrard and Richmond, 1963) to hypothesize that some of the main adverse consequences of major illness may depend upon the *age of onset*. Thus, illness during infancy and early childhood (one to three years) is seen as 'limiting opportunities for self-expression, intensifying maternal control, enhancing passivity and helplessness.' The result is to interfere with the goal of achieving autonomy. In the period from four to six years, the major effect of chronic illness is held to be 'extreme guilt (leading) to excessive inhibition of initiative.' From six to 11 years, the result is 'a sense of inferiority and inadequacy,' while illness during adolescence is thought to 'interfere with the ability to establish clear concepts of role and identity.'

Maddison and Raphael go on to specify certain psychodynamic mechanisms which, they believe, help to understand the social and psychological consequences of chronic illness. These include dependence and regression; restriction of activity; guilt; the nature of childhood thought processes; fear of mutilation; the perception of pain, fear of death; and the pleasures and rewards of illness.

That long-term illness in childhood may ultimately interfere with normal development is a view shared by most investigators. But, like the glass seen by some as half-empty and by others as half-full, some researchers focus more upon those factors which facilitate successful coping, while others concentrate upon the attributes that lead to poor adjustment.

Mattsson (1972) presents a careful analysis of the *adaptational techniques* used by the child and his parents to master the 'negative and distressing emotions' brought about by these illnesses. The techniques described include the use of cognitive functions, motor activity, emotional expression and a range of psychologic defences, *e.g.* denial, isolation and identification. The conclusion reached is that 'the nature of the specific illness appears less influential for a child's successful adaptation than such factors as his developmental level and available coping techniques, the quality of the parent-child relationship, and the family's acceptance.'

Over the past 10 years, one of us (IBP) has been associated with a series of epidemiological surveys designed to determine the extent to which children with *any* chronic physical disorder are prone to secondary emotional sequelae. For this purpose a chronic illness has been defined as 'a physical, usually non-fatal condition which lasted longer than three months in a given year, or necessitated a period of continuous hospitalization of more than one month.' A similar definition has been adopted in the periodic U.S. National Health Surveys, and experience has shown that most conditions meeting this criterion are of very long duration and tend to be permanent.

One of these studies began by analysing data accumulated in the first National Survey of Child Health and Development (Pless and Douglas, 1971). This was a longitudinal study of a representative national sample of all children born during one week in March, 1946 throughout England, Wales and Scotland. The sample, comprising more than 5,000 children, has been examined at intervals, using a variety of measures depending on the age of the cohort at the time of assessment. The first study of those with chronic illnesses was based upon data available at the age of 15 years. All who, prior to that time, had a diagnosis meeting the stated criterion were identified and compared with the remaining 'healthy controls.' A total of 528, representing a cumulative prevalence rate of 111 per thousand children in the cohort, were found to have, or have had, one or more chronic disorders. Twenty per cent were illnesses affecting the respiratory system, such as asthma and bronchitis, 14% were neurological conditions, and 11% were disorders of the musculo-skeletal system. A further 19% involved the special senses — speech, hearing or vision; the remainder included a wide variety of other disorders. Each condition was classified according to the type of disability it produced (*e.g.* motor, sensory or cosmetic); by degree of severity; and by the duration it was expected to last (permanent, indefinite, or temporary). The interrelationships between these classifications were examined and the group as a whole compared with the healthy controls. Although there were more boys than girls in the chronically ill group (57% vs. 51%) ($p. <.01$), the only other significant difference was that the mother's health was more often rated 'fair' or 'poor' for those with illnesses compared with the controls.

Analysis of the educational and behavioural status of this group was subsequently compared with data from the Isle of Wight survey and the Rochester Child Health Studies (Pless and Roghmann, 1971).

The latter were obtained from a 1% random sample of all families with children under 18 years resident in Monroe County in New York State. During the first sample survey, conducted in 1967, parents reported all chronic symptoms observed in the study child during the previous year. Those with symptoms judged by the parent to be 'somewhat' serious or 'very' serious were interviewed a second time the following year, together with a group of presumably healthy children drawn from the same initial sample, but matched for age, sex, race and socio-economic background. A total of 209 children with established chronic illnesses were identified. Although their distribution differs, in terms of category of disorder represented, from both the National Survey and the Isle of Wight Survey, the total prevalence is similar — 119 per thousand with one or more chronic illnesses.

Thus three relatively large population surveys are available from which the frequency of secondary psychosocial consequences can be estimated. In the Rochester study, information obtained from a semi-structured household interview was supplemented by a battery of psychological tests administered directly to the child. Ratings of behaviour were also obtained from the parents and from the child's teachers. In addition, sociometric ratings were constructed, together with information from the school about the child's abilities, achievement and referrals for child guidance, psychological testing or counselling.

The Isle of Wight study showed a much higher rate of specific reading retardation, both for those with neurological disorders (27% were retarded 28 months or more), and those with other chronic disorders (14%), compared with 5% in the controls. The Rochester study revealed a slightly higher frequency of sick children with a significant discrepancy between ability and achievement test scores (35% vs. 31%), and the National Survey showed the same, with the additional finding that rate of retardation was directly related to severity of disorder.

A variety of indices of social functioning were available in the National survey and in the Rochester study. Both revealed a consistent, but statistically non-significant, excess of difficulties among those with chronic illnesses compared with the controls.

In the Isle of Wight Survey, the frequency of psychiatric disturbance was 17% for the chronically ill, compared with 7% for the controls. The National survey data yielded a higher frequency of children with two or more behaviour symptoms (25% vs. 17%); more who were rated nervous, aggressive, or both, by their teachers (39% vs. 31%); and slightly more with self ratings indicative of neuroses (14% vs. 11%).

Initially the behavioural status of the Rochester groups was assessed simply by noting the frequency with which parents reported abnormal symptoms of behaviour in the interview. In the age group 6 — 10, 23% of those with chronic illnesses had 2 or more such symptoms compared with 16% of the controls. In the age group 11 to 15 years, the figures were 30% vs. 13% — suggesting that over time such problems may become more prominent. Further analysis of the data from the Rochester and National survey studies suggests some relationship between maladjustment and type of disorder — those with sensory conditions having the highest rates in both studies. There was also a tendency for those with conditions judged to be permanent to have a slightly higher rate of maladjustment, and a similar, small but direct relationship with severity.

The Rochester studies attempted to take into account the influence of the family unit and more specifically, the quality of family functioning (Pless et al., 1972). To do so an Index was devised based upon responses to questions included in the household interview. In a separate series of trials, the reliability and validity of this Family Functioning Index was established (Pless and Satterwhite, 1973). The index permits the quality of family functioning (reflecting such areas as marital satisfaction, frequency of disagreements, level of happiness, communications, etc.) to be divided into high, medium or low groups depending on the scores obtained.

The results from the entire battery of psychological measures completed by both the chronically ill and healthy controls in the Rochester study were further analysed to enable an overall 'adjustment index' to be calculated. The index incorporates three basic measures — symptom ratings, self-esteem, and teachers' ratings. A high rating (good adjustment) is assigned to those with the 'best' scores on all three measures; a low rating to those with lowest scores on all three (poor adjustment).

Using multiple regression analysis and automatic interaction detection (AID) analysis, it was found that the addition of both family function and family structure scores contributes significantly to the 'prediction' of poor adjustment among the chronically ill. In the age group 6 to 11 years, for example, 23% of children with chronic disorders were found to be poorly adjusted when their family functioning was rated 'good'; compared to 32% of those with 'poor' family functioning scores. In the older age group the discrepancy is even greater: about 17% have poor adjustment scores when family functioning is 'good' compared with 35% when it is 'poor'. Because the data were obtained cross-sectionally, we cannot conclude that, as these figures would suggest, the adjustment of children with chronic illness, in well functioning families, improves over time, while that of children in poorly functioning families worsens — but the possibility exists and warrants further testing.

The AID analysis also suggests — and this is important — that parents' symptom ratings may be best predicted by a combination of the following variables: for the younger age groups, family functioning and health alone; whereas for older children, family functioning, health, self-esteem and sex. Such sophisticated analyses are required because of the complexity of interaction that determines maladjustment.

The major purpose of the Rochester studies has been to try to identify sub-groups among the chronically ill, whose vulnerability or maladjustment 'risk' is highest. To do so, we have incorporated a wider variety of measures than most other studies, while conducting our appraisal, whenever possible, on representative groups of children.

Our conviction that the family plays a key role, has been strengthened by the outcome of an experimental trial, designed to evaluate the efficacy of non-professional family counsellors (Pless and Satterwhite, 1972)(page 201, Section V) We call attention to the study because it was based on the assumption that if we could help the families of these children in any way — through empathetic listening, information about the child's disorder, simple advice, counselling, or by helping the child improve his self-concept — his adjustment would be improved.

To test this premise, six non-professional women were carefully selected and randomly assigned to eight families, four of whom had poor functioning scores and four good functioning scores. All had children with a chronic illness, whose adjustment had been assessed prior to the period of intervention. In a similarly random fashion, a comparable number of high and low functioning families, having children with the same types and severity of chronic disorder, were simultaneously identified to serve as controls. Both experimental group and controls had the psychological tests repeated after a period of one year. The results clearly show that even this simple attention to the family is beneficial: 60% of children in the 55 study families had improved psychological test scores at the end of the year of counselling compared with only 40% of controls who did not receive counselling.

Our more recent studies (Kanthor et al., 1974) examine, in detail, the assistance provided for a family with a severely handicapped child when care is divided between a primary physician (paediatrician or family doctor) and a 'team' of specialists. The study was based on the responses of 44 mothers of children with spina bifida attending a Birth Defects Centre. The results indicate that many of the supportive services related to counselling (even genetic counselling) are not provided under these ciscumstances.

We cite this finding to illustrate further the complexity of the factors involved in promoting good adjustment. In the past, most research has focused on the child and his family, while failing to examine the role of the physician in an objective, critical fashion. There is, however, reason to believe that physicians have much to offer in preventing or ameliorating adjustment difficulties among these children. Regrettably, however, the reverse is also true — health professionals may unwittingly, by sins of omission or commission, contribute to the genesis of these problems.

SCHOLASTIC PERFORMANCE AS AN INDIRECT INDICATOR

As previously noted (p.67, Section III), the effects of illness on school performance may only partially reflect maladjustment. Central nervous system involvement may be alternatively incriminated, as may be frequent or lengthy absences necessitated by the illness or its treatment. Nevertheless, in some cases the postulated effect on self-concept can manifest itself through alterations in school performance, assessed either by classroom behaviour or, more specifically, by scholastic progress in terms of grades or achievement test scores.

The significance of these scores rests upon an assumption of the accuracy with which intellectual abilities can be assessed in childhood. In the past any discrepancy between ability and achievement was commonly viewed as evidence of 'under-achievement.' One explanation for this is the presence of lengthy, disabling illness. More recently, however, the meaning of ability testing and, in particular, the significance of IQ scores has been debated. There has also been concern about assessing achievement in a uniform fashion; more and more school districts have abandoned the use of report cards or standardized achievement testing.

Despite these trends, many studies have attempted to relate effect of illness to both ability and achievement. Several aspects of the issue merit consideration.

Consider, for example, the *origins* of any such adverse effects in relation to scholastic performance. Children who are receiving special education in segregated classes or residential schools may be subject to a standard of instruction inferior to that provided for healthy children in the 'ordinary' school system. Even where the child with chronic illness remains in a 'regular' classroom, the teacher may consciously or unconsciously adjust his demands or his grading of that child's performance, or both, because of the illness. Hence, when these children are compared with their healthy peers in respect of their performance, any difference may reflect the attitudes and behaviour of the child's teacher or school system more than the extent to which 'adjustment' has been affected by the illness.

Our main concern, however, is to tease out what evidence there is for school problems directly attributable to chronic illness.

Of historical interest in this regard is the survey described by Keller (1953). A random sample of all families living in a section of Baltimore, Md. (U.S.) were interviewed over the period from 1938 to 1943. So many changes have occurred in educational and public health practices since then, that it would be misleading to draw any firm conclusions from the findings. The methodology, however, is a model of clarity and simplicity. It begins by dividing the entire sample of 1,209 children between the ages of 6-16 years into two groups — those making 'satisfactory' school progress (based on promotions through regular classrooms) and those whose progress was 'unsatisfactory'. Progress is then related to the presence of a chronic illness, and it is noted that the rate per 1000 population of children with these illnesses is consistently higher in the 'unsatisfactory' than in the 'satisfactory' category. For example, the rate for children with asthma whose school progress was 'unsatisfactory' was 26.9 compared with 17.1 'satisfactory'. For hay fever, the figures were 12.0 and 5.7 respectively, and for heart disease they were 6.0 and 3.4 per 1000. In the group of children with 'other' chronic disease (*i.e.* excluding mental retardation and behaviour problems), the rate was 32.9 per 1000 with 'unsatisfactory' progress! Even when other social factors were taken into account, most of these striking differences remained.

Scholastic achievement of children with central nervous system disorders
The studies originating from the Isle of Wight Survey, dealing with CNS disorders and their effects on education, are perhaps the most rigorous and systematic ever to be recorded. The main study had centred only upon children aged 10-12 years, but a special neuropsychiatric study included all school-age children (Rutter and Graham, 1970). Broadly speaking two groups are considered — those with known mental retardation and those assumed, for the most part, to be of normal intelligence. Although retarded children can also 'underachieve' if ability is taken into consideration, our concern here is primarily with those having chronic illnesses of the CNS which do not necessarily result in retardation.

Epileptic children are one such group who, as noted

previously, have a normal level of intelligence provided the epilepsy is uncomplicated by other neurological dysfunction. In a paper devoted to the enigmas surrounding educational attainment in epileptic children, Yule (1973) draws attention to the relatively few well-conceived, systematic studies on the subject. He asserts that 'very few studies comment on the educational attainment of (epileptic) children, although there are many clinical impressions that epileptic children underachieve at school.' Several possible factors are discussed; brain dysfunction, school absence, the effect of anticonvulsant drugs, and the educational expectations of parents, teachers and the children themselves. Drawing upon the Isle of Wight data, Yule showed that although the average IQ of children with uncomplicated epilepsy was 102 (on the WISC), they were reading about 12 months behind the level expected for children of comparable chronological age. He notes that this finding is in accord with that of Ounsted *et al.* (1966) who found children in their clinic to be 'academic failures in spite of good intelligence.'

The results from the Isle of Wight survey further showed that 18% of children with uncomplicated epilepsy were retarded in reading by as much as 24 months or more, after age and IQ are both taken into account. Compare this with a similar degree of reading retardation in only 6.8% of children in the control group. The finding cannot be explained by absence from school alone, and hence points to brain dysfunction involving those specific abilities concerned in learning to read, or other psychological mechanisms governing self-perception.

The latter possibility receives some support from the work of Green and Hartlage (1971, 1972) who relate underachievement to parental over-protection and lower educational aspirations. In their first study, the Wide Range Achievement Test (along with several other measures) was administered to children with epilepsy and the results compared with normative values after correction for age and intelligence. Although the children with epilepsy were found to be 'better developed in self-direction than their non-epileptic controls,' they compared poorly on all other measures. Specifically, it was found that whereas children with epilepsy were at appropriate academic grade placements, they were 'from one to two years below expectancy on academic skill levels' with reading being the least affected (13 months below) and arithmetic the most affected (21 months below). They concluded 'in general it appears that the epileptic children do not measure up to academic skill levels commensurate with their abilities' and suggested that 'parental expectancies may be lower . . . and would be compatible with the possibility that the epileptic child is hindered . . . (because) he is not expected to perform at the rate which would be expected if he were not epileptic.' The authors suggest that 'it may be of value to emphasize their assets and responsibilities rather than dwelling on the limiting aspects of their condition.'

Among children with more serious and extensive disorders involving the nervous system, such as cerebral palsy, it is not surprising that school performance is often found to be very poor. Taking the group of children with organic brain disorders of any kind together, Rutter et al. (1970) found 26.5% with specific reading retardation of at least 28 months compared with only 5.8% controls who were similarly retarded. (Since this measure is calculated 'on the basis of the level of reading expected in terms of the child's chronological age and WISC IQ,' the results cannot be attributed to mental subnormality alone). Similarly, in Bowley's study of 65 children with cerebral palsy (1967), although only 37% were below average intelligence, more than one-half were school failures and only 11 were able to transfer to ordinary schools.

Mention should also be made of the intriguing work reported by Smith and McWilliams (1968) concerning children with speech problems due to cleft palate. One hundred and thirty-six children between the ages of three and nine years were studied using the Illinois Test of Psycholinguistic Abilities. At all age levels the children with clefts had depressed results in the areas of language sampled. The weaknesses were greatest in the areas of vocal and gestural expression and visual memory. These findings are difficult to interpret. They suggest a general visuo-motor deficit which may be related to early deprivation in motor development due to early surgical treatment, or to the 'shyness, dependency, rigidity, inhibition and general lack of affect often attributed to cleft children.'

Several other studies have been reported concerning children with disorders involving the special senses — speech, hearing, and vision. Alberman *et al.* (1971) studied the educational performance of children with strabismus (squints). Data was obtained from the National Child Development Study comprising more than 15,000 children born in 1958. Of these, 482 were identified as having a squint by the age of seven years, and, after excluding cerebral palsy or subnormality, the remaining 478 were compared with 12,904 controls. In addition to the cosmetic defect of the squint itself, the results show that visual acuity is diminished as is the academic performance of these children. Significant differences emerged between the scores of the squint cases and the controls on teachers' ratings of reading skills, but not on an arithmetic test. Many of these differences remained even after excluding those judged to be 'clumsy' (presumably evidence of neurologic dysfunction), and those of low birth weight.

Douglas *et al.* (1967), drawing upon data from an earlier national cohort study, describe analyses which show that short-sighted (myopic) children attain *better* achievement test results than children of 'normal' vision, despite the two groups being similar on non-verbal intelligence tests. The short-sighted group is characterized by being more hard-working and more attentive in class, having many academic hobbies and taking relatively little interest in sports. Generally, they are successful at school and have high ambitions for further education and employment. These results raise fascinating questions about cause and effect relationships. The authors hypothesize that 'families with a history of short-sight have, over the generations, acquired academic interests and a high valuation of non-manual or professional employment that are passed on to the children.'

We have already commented upon the relatively poor academic achievement of deaf adolescents and adults. Studies by Vernon (1967a, b) and Levine (1951) show that these achievements are further compromised when deafness is associated with prematurity or the rubella syndrome. In both studies IQ scores are depressed significantly below those expected for deaf populations and, in general, educational performance reflects this further handicap.

The study by Rubin *et al.* (1973) is but one of many demonstrating that prematurity alone results in severe educational disadvantages. Specifically, Rubin's study showed that males with low birth weights and children of both sexes who were 'small-for-dates' had a significantly higher incidence of school problems warranting special school placement and special school services than did full birth weight, full term controls. The low birth weight children also had lower scores on academic achievement at the age of seven years.

Scholastic achievement of children with disorders not involving the central nervous system

Earlier studies of abnormalities in physique reviewed by Barker *et al.* (1953) had examined the psychological correlates of extreme deviations in height and weight. It is only recently, however, and through the studies of Money and his colleagues, that interest in this group of children has been revived. In the first of a series of papers describing the psychology of dwarfism, Pollitt and Money (1964) show that although prior to treatment with growth hormone the 15 children studied were generally of normal intelligence, their school achievement as rated by parents and school personnel was uniformly at or below average. Eight of the children were noted to lack interest in their school work and to have poor study habits. A later report, however, shows significant improvements in school performance resulting from therapy with growth hormone.

These findings are likely to be attributable not to physiological factors alone, but also to psychological mechanisms. Donner and Elton (1973) studied 28 children of short stature, of whom one-half had growth hormone deficiency. The group had IQ scores in the normal range, but, of those aged seven or older, nearly 50% were retarded in their reading achievement by more than 20 months. Parents were concerned about both their school functioning and their social functioning. It is reasonable to postulate that the two may be related. The authors comment, 'It would be obviously ridiculous to attribute poor school achievement, in a boy whose medical condition means that he is intellectually limited, to his short stature, but it would be just as unwise to ignore the effects of nutritional deficiencies that also occur in many short stature children.'

It is stressed that because of the perfectly normal appearance of these children apart from their stature, it is hard not to treat them as if they were much younger. 'Short stature children have a limited number of available social roles and those they do adopt tend to perpetuate social relationships that make it difficult for them to behave in a way that is consistent with their age. Some of the children adapted by becoming withdrawn and isolated from their peers; others clearly preferred the company of younger children.' The authors suggest that when events conspire to make a child behave in a way appropriate for a younger child, this is germane to the finding that such children, as a group, appear to function poorly at school.

Haemophilia is another disorder which does not involve the nervous system. Apart from the observations by Katz, already noted, a study by Olch (1971a) of 45 children under the age of 21 shows that, despite 'high average' range of intelligence, both grade discrepancies and achievement test discrepancies were significantly lowered. Of importance is the finding that these discrepancies increase with age, suggesting that the impact of the illness on performance increases over time. It does not appear, however, that this can be explained by the cumulative effect of absences, since there was no correlation between low achievement and poor attendance. As might be expected, intelligence, socio-economic level and certain personality attributes were related to school achievement.

In a large-scale study of physically disabled high school students by Allen (1967), more than 2,000 with such conditions as restricted use of a limb, hearing loss, partial blindness, and a variety of other disorders, were matched with healthy controls for the purpose of comparing their vocational aspirations and expectations. Highly significant differences were found between the two groups in the direction of lower cumulative grade point averages for those with impairments.

For children with a range of chronic physical disorders not involving the nervous system, the most comprehensive and well-designed survey of educational achievement is that undertaken by Rutter *et al.* (1970). No less than 14% of the 114 children between the ages of 10-12 were significantly retarded in reading compared with 5.4% of control children. In this case, the retardation was correlated with the high school absence rate. It is noteworthy, moreover, that children with disorders other than asthma and eczema were found to be of lower intelligence. Although this finding may be simply related to the small numbers involved (42), it was in this group that the rate of absence was highest. The authors conclude, 'It may be that these children's very frequent absence from school had a slightly retarding effect on intelligence development as well as on scholastic progress.' However, the point is made that, 'It is not that the children have had one prolonged absence from school. Most children can compensate for that without too much difficulty. These children have had repeated short absences with all that means in terms of discouragement and lowering of morale and confidence. The effects on the children's work attitudes may well be as important as the actual school time missed.'

The effects of chronic illness on intelligence

From what is known about the basic nature of intelligence in children, there is little evidence that, apart from retardation due to organic brain damage, intellectual development should be impaired as a consequence of chronic illness. Indeed, a number of studies emphasize that intelligence is normally distributed among these children. For example, Ack *et al.* (1961) showed that the IQ scores of 38 children with diabetes were similar to those of their randomly selected siblings, and bore no relation to duration of illness except among children whose diabetes had begun before the age of five years. Pollitt and Money (1964), in their study of dwarfs, demonstrated that IQ scores were normally distributed; this has also been shown by Goetzinger and Proud (1966) in their review of the effects of severe early deafness. Similarly, Gayton and Friedman (1973), reviewing the psychological aspects of cystic fibrosis, concluded that 'it would appear that CF children are not significantly different from normal children in regard to the distribution of IQ.' (Only one of the studies reviewed commented on *academic* functioning — noting considerable educational retardation even among those children of average or above average intelligence (Lawler *et al.*, 1966)).

There are, nevertheless, many reports that show the extent to which IQ scores are lowered in association with chronic physical disorder. The presumption of a causal relationship is strengthened on occasion by an increase in score following some improvement in the child's condition. Thus the studies of Linde *et al.* (1970), Honzik *et al.* (1969) and Landtmann *et al.* (1960, 1968), each relating to children with congenital heart disease, all document some improvement in IQ scores following corrective surgery. In the first of these studies the mean IQ improved in both the acyanotic and cyanotic patients as well as in controls, but following covariance analysis, improvement was found chiefly in cyanotic children after operation though not in the inoperable group. Changes in the acyanotic group were insignificant. In Honzik's report, the changes were related to sex and to component verbal and performance sections of the WISC.

Reviewing 50 years' research on the intellectual ability of patients with epilepsy, Tarter (1972) concluded that 'unselected epileptics exhibit a mean IQ slightly lower than the population norm.' Those with symptomatic or secondary epilepsy have lower scores than idiopathic epileptics and institutionalized subjects have lower scores still. The evidence reviewed also suggests that that degree of deterioration is directly related to premorbid IQ, to type of seizure (major seizures being more destructive than petit mal), age of onset, number of seizures and total duration of the illness.

Francis-Williams (1965) in a similarly extensive review of the intelligence of children with cerebral palsy, states that approximately 48% of those who are testable have IQs below 70. She stresses the inadvisability of using one test only 'since they suffer from so many handicaps which affect cognitive functioning.' In particular, the performance scale of the WISC is likely to be especially misleading because it involves so many timed tests requiring motor coordination.

There is long-standing debate as to whether children with muscular dystrophy are truly retarded or whether their frequent academic difficulties are secondary to this distressing, progressive disease. The issue is complicated by the finding that scholastic achievement is 'frequently poor even in the earliest school years when . . . muscle weakness is relatively mild.' This observation suggests that there may be a common genetic or other underlying factor affecting intellectual function independent of the basic motor neurone defect. The literature is fairly evenly divided on whether retardation, when present, is primary or secondary.

In an attempt to determine whether boys with PMD* function at an intellectual level significantly different from the general population Worden and Vignos (1962) tested 38 patients between the ages of four and 17 years (mean age of 11 years) using Form M of the Stanford-Binet. The average IQ score was 83, ranging from 46 to 134. More important, only three children scored above 110 and 26 scored below 90. Thus, there was a definite downward shift in the distribution curve. (Reading and arithmetic achievement test scores were consistent with these ability levels.) There was, however, no correlation with severity of disease, nor with its duration. Nor could the scores be attributed to family factors since siblings had significantly greater scores, average 110. Chronicity of disorder was no more convincing an explanation because 36 matched children with diabetes had a mean IQ of 107 and another group of more severely disabled children with myotonia congenita had a mean IQ of 118. The authors conclude that the 'mean IQ is significantly below normal in children with PMD' and that the cause of this depression is unlikely to be emotional but more probably related to metabolic abnormalities in the CNS.

Because children with meningomyelocele (spina bifida) also have hydrocephalus, it is not surprising that their intellectual functioning is frequently impaired. It has been estimated that about one-half of children with this disorder who survive to school age have normal intelligence and most of these could, if circumstances allowed, function in normal schools (Stephen, 1963; Badell-Ribera et al., 1966; Laurence and Tew, 1967). A study by Scherzer and Gardner (1971) examines 14 school-age children using a battery of psychological tests of both intelligence and personality. The results of intelligence testing showed eight children with full scale scores between 87 and

* PMD — progressive muscle dystrophy.

117 and the remainder to be retarded, including three with scores below 51. In this study, hydrocephalus was not predictive of intelligence but in several cases it was mild and spontaneously arrested. Although the results of the Vineland Test of Social Maturity generally paralleled IQ scores, in four cases the social quotient was 15 or more points lower. The authors suggest that this 'probably reflects the tendency of parents to over-protect . . . thus unnecessarily limiting their development of social maturity.'

To summarize, where the potential effects of chronic illness on IQ have been examined, scores in some groups of cases have been found to be significantly depressed. This is to be expected in disorders involving the brain, but is difficult to explain for many other conditions. In both groups, however, the results must be interpreted cautiously. Psychologists readily acknowledge the difficulty of accurately assessing children with gross motor or sensory disorders. Furthermore, the validity of the measures used is questionable because of the restrictions on day-to-day activities imposed by many childhood illnesses. Thus, the significance of findings remains problematic. On the one hand, taken at face value, they suggest that a chronic illness can truly result in retardation or pseudo-retardation. On the other hand, such an interpretation is held by some to be misleading since it does not accurately reflect the child's innate intellectual ability and this is what measures of intelligence are intended to describe.

PSYCHOLOGICAL MALADJUSTMENT IN SPECIFIC CHRONIC ILLNESSES

A. Disorders of the central nervous system

Poliomyelitis, although now rarely seen in Western countries, served for many years as a prototype of central nervous system disorder yielding significant psychosocial sequelae. In an important early contribution along these lines, Seidenfeld (1948) begins by stating the research issue in the following terms: 'It may be held that any disease . . . of sufficient duration . . . which actually alters the child's capacity to live in a manner to which he has become accustomed is likely to produce alterations in his adjustment sufficient in proportion to tax his capacity to make new adjustments.' Reviewing earlier psychological studies of children with polio (beginning with a report in 1930), Seidenfeld was unable to draw any firm conclusions about the extent of problems in adjustment among them.

In his own study of 110 cases, ranging in age from 9 to 15 years, he employed an early form of the California Test of Personality. Only 22% had scores below the 50th percentile — suggesting either 'a minimum of emotional and personality problems' among his subjects, or insensitivity of the test. Through further analysis, however, Seidenfeld found evidence of a 'remarkable degree of "likemindedness" in responses'. By using selected items, he showed that those whose disability was 'apparent' were, in fact, responding in a fashion indicative of maladjustment. He concluded, 'It seems highly probable that to the extent that the presence of a physical handicap represents an actual restricting element in the life of the patient, it is altogether likely that adjustment will be less adequate than desired, and feelings against one's environment will be present.'

These findings are in contrast to several earlier studies (*e.g.* Kammerer, 1940; Gates, 1946), in which the 'apparent normalcy' of response to objective tests predominated. (Seidenfeld's major contribution in our view was to recognize the limitations in design and procedures used in his own and other studies, calling attention to the existence of sub-groups among the chronically ill who are most seriously affected.)

In succeeding years, attention shifted to other disorders such as cerebral palsy once it became clear that many more children with this condition were going to survive. Mitchell (1971) lucidly expresses the philosophy underlying this growing interest. 'Greater understanding of the natural history of cerebral palsy gained by following affected individuals from early childhood through into adult life has taught us that the ultimate handicap is related as much to the consequences of having a disability as to the degree and type of cerebral palsy. Perhaps most important is the effect of being handicapped on personality and emotional development, but also to be considered is the impact on the educational achievement of the child produced by the motor disorder, associated sensory, intellectual and other disabilities, and frequent absences from school for treatment or because of intercurrent illness. The combined result . . . is all too often progressive social deprivation and isolation which in time becomes the greatest handicap.'

Ingram's study (page 84) provides evidence of the truth of this prediction, calling particular attention to the role of personality problems in the poor employment patterns so often noted. Bowley (1972) also found that more than half the children studied had emotional reactions regarded as 'abnormal' (based on a teachers' check list of symptoms) and about one in five had social maturity scores below their mental ages. Apart from severity of handicap, the latter were related to parental over-protection, excessive pressure or insecurity. Such attitudes may, to some extent, account for differences in parental assessment of the child's abilities compared with those made by professional workers — differences which, on the whole, err on the side of over-estimates (Keith and Markie, 1969; Jensen and Kogan, 1962) (see page 191, Section V).

Relatively few investigators have attempted to assess the adjustment of children with cerebral palsy using projective techniques. One exception is the work of Abercrombie and Tyson (1966) in which the Draw-a-Man Test was used to estimate mental age, but additionally, to assess disordered body-image. The results were so totally inconclusive that the authors advise against using this procedure for this purpose.

Even fewer studies have employed objective observations as a means of evaluating the child's emotional state. In a carefully designed field study to assess the degree of disturbance brought about by surgery, 50 children with cerebral palsy were systematically observed pre- and post-operatively (Reynell, 1965). In spite of formidable difficulties, the author succeeded in making a continuous written record of observations of factors such as responsiveness, attention, emotional state, pain, fatigue and fear. Patients were followed for nine months following surgery. The trends observed were surprisingly consistent, with marked behavioural disturbance characterizing the majority of children. Although the results are of limited value in establishing the frequency of persisting maladjustment, they clearly demonstrate the applicability of this technique — and its limitations.

Hersov (1963) has reviewed the work of others relating to emotional factors in cerebral palsy. Several reports are cited showing a high frequency of emotional disturbance (*e.g.* Dunsdon, 1952; Floyer, 1955; Crothers and Paine, 1959), and the importance of parental attitudes is repeatedly emphasized. The work of Shere and Kastenbaum (1966) is of particular importance in this respect. Through systematic interviews and observations of mother-child interaction in 13 children with cerebral palsy, they were able to document the extent to which 'individual and family dynamics play an important role in the cognitive development of handicapped children', and note that 'frequently the dynamics of interaction serve to inhibit rather than facilitate development.' Several important recommendations stem from this study to help guide programmes of preventive intervention. In essence, the authors urge that guidance begin at the time of diagnosis; that special attention be given to the mothers' expectations that 'little or no pleasure will be forthcoming from interactions with the (disabled) child'; and finally, that mothers must be helped to achieve a realistic view of their children. (It is of interest that the emphasis throughout this paper, and most others, is exclusively on the role of mothers — fathers are rarely, if ever, mentioned.)

Similar emphasis is placed on the crucial role of parental attitudes in the genesis of adjustment problems so frequently encountered among epileptic children. As Crowther (1967) states, 'The epileptic child is a victim of his environment. Well-meaning parents and friends are frequently over-protective . . . the natural tendency is to restrict the child lest serious injury might result. Some of these misgivings are legitimate . . . However, the benefit to the child may be outweighed by the effect of these restrictions on his emotional development.'

Although much the same points are made by Ireton (1969), certain implications for the physician stand out more clearly. 'The reaction of the child and his family to the fact of seizures, both in crisis and in the long run, has as much to do with the physician's ability to identify with and communicate with parents and child, as it does with drug management.' Ireton suggests that many of the adjustment problems of children with seizures might be prevented by comprehensive medical care. He cites, in particular, the experiences of Baus *et al.* (1958) and Defries and Bowder (1952) in the use of group sessions as one means of accomplishing this goal.

Richardson and Friedman (1974) interviewed 17 adolescents with epilepsy to determine areas they themselves viewed as special problems. Major psychosocial difficulties were found in 13 of the families, but the nature of the problems as reported by the patients differed somewhat from those reported by their parents. The teenagers emphasized relations with their peers as a focus of concern whereas parents were chiefly preoccupied with behaviour, *e.g.* depression. The authors point out that 'schools are afraid of sick children, especially those with epilepsy . . .' and several means of improving this situation are proposed.

In addition to the literature summarized by the Epilepsy Foundation (1967), much of which includes both behavioural disturbance and its therapy, two other recent publications deal with the problems of epileptic children in considerable detail. Bagley's book, *The Social Psychology of the Epileptic Child* (1971), incorporates a comprehensive review of psychiatric aspects. While recognizing that the methodology of many studies is open to criticism, because of doubtfully representative sampling, absence of control groups, and dubious validity of the measures employed to rate disturbance, the figures quoted for the prevalence of personality disorders range from 12% to 60%. Bagley finds fairly general agreement that the main types of disorder include a neurotic pattern, aggressive and antisocial behaviour, overactive or hyperkinetic behaviour and mental defect. Although careful to point out that the findings are often in conflict, he draws attention to the links that have been demonstrated between personality disturbance and brain damage, intelligence, sex, body build, parental reactions, nature of the fits and the role of environmental factors.

In his own controlled study, Bagley compared 83 disturbed epileptics with similarly disturbed children but without epilepsy; and 35 epileptics without behaviour disorder with matched controls who had both epilepsy *and* disturbed behaviour. The results confirm the importance of social factors (disturbed environment, family pathology and neurosis in family members) in the aetiology of maladjustment. A subsequent section similarly stresses the significance of parental attitudes but he notes that their potency is affected by how far they interact with adverse environmental factors and the type of seizures manifested. Bagley suggests that 'The hypothesis of interaction *i.e.* that many different factors have a partial influence on the final behavioural outcome in epilepsy, may help to explain some of the apparently contradictory findings which have emerged in some studies.'

Such is the multiplicity of factors identified in his studies, that the author's recommendations for improving services for these children focus predictably upon the integration of medical, social and educational agencies — particularly the hospital and the school. Likewise, Bagley argues strongly in favour of an integrated approach to the understanding of human behaviour, drawing equally upon sociological, psychological and biological knowledge and theories.

A strikingly similar report, reaching much the same conclusions, is described by Goldin and his colleagues in their book, *The Rehabilitation of the Young Epileptic: Dimensions and Dynamics* (1971). They begin by accepting that 'The epileptic is prone to psychosocial maladjustment . . .' and that this may result in '. . . a pervasive subacute type of dependency which may interfere with the development of adequate coping mechanisms.' (p. 8). Thus the purpose of the study is 'to describe and assess the juvenile epileptic's level of psychosocial functioning within the familial, educational, recreational and vocational systems, and to make recommendations which are fundamental to his rehabilitation.'

The work was carried out by sending a questionnaire to the parents of a sample of 571 epileptics traced through physicians, hospitals, schools and state rehabilitation agencies. Of the 231 questionnaires returned, 203 were usable and were supplemented in 25 cases by personal interviews. The respondents were divided into two groups — those with epilepsy alone (n = 148) and those with epilepsy and another disability, such as mental retardation or some physical disorder (n = 55).

Differences between these two groups were noted with respect to relations with siblings, restriction of family activities, leisure time activities, and general adjustment. In all cases, those with additional disabilities compared unfavourably in each of these areas. It is worth noting, however, that, overall, one-third of the group were judged to be poorly adjusted psychologically, on the basis of various indices of daily activities.

Although there was no attempt to measure self-concept directly, its central role is repeatedly stressed. 'The influence of self-concept upon adjustment and achievement is paramount. An individual's self-concept is highly influenced by the acceptance of significant others in his milieu. In the case of an epileptic child, rejection by family members, particularly siblings, will serve to weaken the child's self-concept by accentuating and reinforcing already existing feelings of deviance, unworthiness and guilt. The resultant poor self-image may engender counter hostility in the epileptic toward his sibs . . . On the other hand, it is altogether possible that the child may have a poor self-image in spite of good acceptance by his parents and sibs. In this case, it may be his perception of the community's evaluation of him which is the critical factor. Nevertheless, family acceptance and warmth can mitigate these feelings of inadequacy and defectiveness.'

In general, we agree with the authors' description of the dynamics of maladjustment, although regrettably their data provide little direct support for their interpretations. Nevertheless, the recommendations they make for promoting the rehabilitation of these children are based as much upon their direct findings as upon the more liberal interpretation of their meaning. Their major emphasis is on the need for earlier, more comprehensive and more continuous counselling (p. 69). (Forty-three per cent of 197 respondents reported having received some professional counselling for their child.) They point to the value of involving *both* parents, with the goal of helping them achieve 'awareness of the effects of their relationship with the child upon his adjustment to life, and the role which family factors play in this adjustment.' Wisely, the authors recognize the need 'to help parents cope with their own feelings' but emphasize that to do so 'the particular professional discipline of the counsellor is not important.' They stress, however, the need for special training for counsellors; for experimentation with group counselling; for more use of integrated social and educational resources; and for more awareness by physicians of the social and emotional factors involved, and of the network of community agencies available to provide services for these children.

Their concluding comment echoes a theme repeatedly encountered in our review of the literature: 'The findings of this study reinforce what has long been known — the disabling potential of epilepsy in children is as much psychosocial as it is physical. Perhaps more so. Medical services for the young epileptic have advanced encouragingly. Social and vocational services have lagged behind. The need for comprehensive community planning in this area is crucial.'

B. Special senses

Children with disorders of speech, hearing or vision are likely to become emotionally disturbed or experience difficulties in social relationships for many reasons. Each of these conditions imposes a major barrier in the path of direct communication with other children and with their parents. Blindness and deafness are potent forces influencing reactions in others, in part because of their 'visibility.' There is no way in which a child can conceal the fact that he cannot see or hear, and the same holds true for imperfect speech.

In addition to the strong reactions they evoke in others and the enormity of the loss and deprivation they represent for the child himself, these disorders have an additional potential for emotional disturbance through their links with scholastic achievement. The frustration of being obliged to learn without the aid of sight or hearing, or of trying to communicate despite severe and embarrassing speech disorder, is one obvious reason for scholastic underachievement even allowing for the most advanced special educational techniques. Moreover, because the basis of each of these conditions lies in the central nervous system (in most instances), associated learning problems of a perceptual nature may co-exist, adding to the burden.

Not surprisingly, research into the psychological consequences of blindness and deafness has been extensive. In the case of speech, the major interest has focused upon psychological antecedents for conditions that do not have a clear organic basis, *e.g.* cleft palate. Yet the majority of reports have neither appeared in the general medical nor in the psychological literature and hence, both interest in, and knowledge about these conditions is extremely limited. Although the average physician is unlikely to have much experience of children with these disorders, we believe they represent an important prototype of one aspect of chronic illness and one that merits increasing medical attention. Moreover, the partially blind and partially deaf are seen more frequently in an average practice, as are children with less severe speech difficulties. A considerable body of evidence now points to the possibility that it is these less severely effected children whose disability is 'marginal', among whom psychological problems may be the most frequent (see page 171).

Parmelee (1966), Wolff (1966) and Cohen (1966) each describe some of the basic ways in which blindness affects children's development, particularly in the cognitive sphere. The point is made that many blind children arrive at school 'either emotionally disturbed or intellectually unprepared.' The need for more touch, sound and movement stimulation is emphasized along with the need for more independence and more contact with sighted nursery school children. The basic issue, however, is the relative importance of visual input in cognitive and personality development. The fact that blindness represents reduced stimulation is often linked to the development of stereotyped activity in some form which adds to its stigmatizing potential. This behaviour also contributes to the distress of mothers, many of whom are already experiencing difficulty in developing an attachment to their infants because of the deprivation they encounter in the child's limited responses.

The work described by Cohen represents one of the better studies in relation to emotional adjustment because of its longitudinal nature. Although its major emphasis is on intellectual functioning (most children with lowered intelligence scores had other physiological impairments besides blindness), some observations are made on emotional functioning. Cohen states that it is secondary to unfavourable reactions from others, especially from the parents, and that this leads to distortion of normal social relationships. Parental pain and guilt create anxiety and depression. Blindness from birth 'may have less consequence for the child's own psychological self-concept, once formed, but children born blind tend to be more affected by other people's attitudes towards them'. The work of Cowen and his colleagues (p.116) raises some doubt about Cohen's categorical conclusion that 'There is no evidence whatsoever that partial sight is a worse handicap than total blindness because of a conflict in whether the child behaves as a blind or sighted child.' Despite disagreement on this score, there is overall acceptance of the emphasis placed on 'good general intelligence as the key factor to successful adjustment.'

In support of this position, Hardy (1968) has shown a significant *inverse* relationship between verbal intelligence and anxiety scores among blind students, 122 of whom were studied by using a specially adapted Anxiety Scale for the Blind. It is also of import, as Hardy found, that anxiety tends to increase with age.

Kellmer-Pringle (1964), in her extensive review, demonstrated how most earlier research into emotional adjustment of the blind had reached conflicting conclusions. She attributed this to wide variations in methodological adequacy. A major approach to the study of blind children was inspired by Burlingham (1961), based on psychoanalytic principles. Such investigations are invariably insightful in observations but these cannot be regarded as scientifically conclusive. Dinnage (1972) summarizes the findings from this extended series of reports by stating 'There is general agreement that emotional deprivation and rejection are more important in the histories of these disturbed children than the sensory deprivation, but it seems that while partially sighted children might have the resources to develop normally to some extent, blind children are especially vulnerable through their inability to understand and protest. Withdrawn, autistic behaviour is the form of psychiatric disturbance most frequently described.'

On the other hand, Cowen *et al.* (1961) found few significant differences between blind students at a residential school, those living at home and sighted matched controls when tested with a variety of objective and projective measures. The differences that were found were neither consistent nor systematic, with the exception of more frequent signs of maladjustment among the partially sighted compared with the totally blind. Good adjustment was related to parental acceptance, an element of normalization in the parents' attitudes, and to social class.

Another of the few studies on blind children in which controls were included and which employed objective tests is that of Zahran (1965). The subjects were pupils at residential schools for the blind (n = 50) and were matched by age, sex, social background and IQ, with healthy children. In addition to a structured interview, the test battery included the Junior Maudsley Personality Inventory, a sentence completion test, and a semantic differential. The only important significant difference found was in the self-evaluation responses on the semantic differential indicating 'less self-confidence' and 'less confidence in the future' among the blind students

Although studies on the adjustment of *deaf* children have been equally, if not more prolific, there remains a dearth of systematic psychiatric studies. Simpson's (1964) extensive survey of 359 children in schools for the deaf suggests a rate of maladjustment of about 12%, while Graham and Rutter (1970) found that 15% of the 13 deaf children identified in the Isle of Wight survey had a psychiatric disorder (compared with 6.6% in the control population of 10 − 11-year-olds).

Based on his study of 51 deaf children, aged five to 14, pupils at a residential school in Britain, Williams (1970) concluded 'that deafness is not a cause of maladjustment but that the inability to communicate is an additional stress to the constellation of environmental and inherent factors which lead to behaviour disorder in childhood.' Two findings are worthy of special attention: the first, that some 40% of the group were classed as having antisocial disorders and 20% as psychotic; the second, that there were fewer disturbed children in the group with the most severe hearing loss than among those with more moderate impairment.

Williams also calls attention to the 'extraordinary, unwelcome and unlikely finding' that earlier diagnosis is associated with a more severe degree of handicap. Several explanations are offered including the possible effect that 'early diagnosis has on parental and other environmental influences.'

In an earlier paper, Williams (1968) reasons that the increased incidence of maladjustment in handicapped children is a 'disturbance of the cybernetic relationship between the handicapped child and his environment as a consequence of the specific handicap.' Faulty behaviour patterns may be learned because the nature of the handicap fails to stimulate the parent to make appropriate responses to the child, or alternatively, stimulates the child's caretakers to inappropriate responses. This hypothesis is consistent with the somato-psychological model described in Section I (page 24).

These findings fit with those of Vernon (1967a, b) in his studies of post-rubella deaf children and cases of deafness associated with prematurity. They are also in accord with the work of Vegely et al. (1968) who used the California Test of Personality in examining 53 deaf children. The results, compared with the published test norms, showed that all median subtest scores except one fell below the 50th percentile. Although the authors recognize the limitations of applying to these children a test standardized on a normal (hearing) population, they argue that it is nevertheless applicable. They hypothesize that 'even after revision of items and test norms, deaf children as a group would continue to show poorer adjustment'; adding that 'the possibility exists that this measured poorer personal adjustment may be a life-long characteristic of the hearing-impaired population.'

The work of Goetzinger and his colleagues (1964, 1966) also indicates the extent to which even those with small perceptive hearing losses are further handicapped by psychosocial problems. 'The incidence of comments from teachers, stressing poor work habits, poor attitudes and emotional variability, was much higher for the hearing loss subjects than for those with normal hearing.' Studies of this group on deaf adolescents, using the SORT (see page 56), revealed a number of significantly different responses between the subjects and normal controls, indicative of maladjustment in several specific areas.

In an attempt to avoid some of the pitfalls of earlier studies (because they had relied upon paper and pencil tests of questionable validity for children with language incapacities), Reivich and Rothrock (1972) employed a Behaviour Problem Checklist (see page 39) completed by the child's teacher. A total of 327 children were included, ranging in age from six to 20 years, all of whom were in a state school for the deaf. This study is important because the instrument chosen is one of the better measures of this kind, and secondly, the analysis of the results employed an advanced statistical technique (factor analysis). Rather than answering the question of frequency of maladjustment overall, the study clearly identifies two factors — isolation and communication problems — that appear unique to children with deafness. The population studied had conduct, personality and immaturity scores that were considerably higher than the mean scores reported for healthy children of similar ages.

Two other recent studies must be cited. The first, by Rodda (1970), is of importance because of its size and the use of an objective measure of adjustment — The Bristol Social Adjustment Guide. Two hundred and thirty school-leavers on whom ratings were obtained, showed a higher, but not significant number of symptoms of maladjustment when compared with norms for hearing children. The symptoms found were chiefly neurotic and withdrawal in character, rather than aggressive or antisocial, and were negatively related to intelligence and social class. Again there is the finding that the partially hearing had special difficulties unlike those of the totally deaf (see page 171, Section V).

This issue of the 'marginal' status of partial deafness was discussed in some detail by Sussman in the proceedings of a National Research Conference on Behavioural Aspects of Deafness (1965). As Sussman puts it, 'Another concept, of special significance to the consideration of disability which is not immediately visible to the observer is that of marginality. (This) is a term used in the race and nationality relations studies to describe the individual who belongs to two cultural worlds . . . he is on the edge, both socially and psychologically . . . A number of studies suggest that persons who are totally deaf may make a better adjustment than the hard of hearing because they know that they cannot hear, and unlike the hard of hearing do not have to worry about the limits of their ability to communicate via the auditory apparatus.' Sussman believes that marginality is more frequently a problem among those who become deaf later in life since those with early deafness can establish socialization patterns that are adequate to their needs.

The second recent study of importance is that of Schlesinger and Meadow (1972). This book reports the findings of a detailed survey of 49 preschool deaf children and 20 hearing 'controls', focusing attention on the constellation of levels of deafness, communication facility and parental attitudes and behaviours. A second part of the study involves school-age children, some in residential schools and some attending day schools, comparing those whose parents are deaf with those that have normal hearing. For this part of the study, a total of 58 pairs of deaf residential school children, half of whose parents were deaf, were included along with 74 day-school deaf children. The groups were assessed with a teacher rating scale, tests of lip reading skill, and a standard achievement test. In addition, an attempt was made to examine the children's self-image and to identify their reference groups. As have so many other investigators, Schlesinger and Meadow refer to Cooley's 'looking-glass self' notion which emphasizes the degree to which self-appraisal is a reflection of the appraisals of others. Accordingly the self-image test was 'designed to measure the ways in which the deaf child interpreted the ideas (other people) had about him, as well as his own self-appraisal.' Interestingly, the residential group with deaf parents scored significantly higher on this test than either those with hearing parents or deaf children in day schools with hearing parents (62% vs. 46%). A specially devised Index of Family Climate also proved to be an important predictor of high self-image scores for children in two of these groups. For example, for residential students with deaf parents, the self-image scores were high in 75% of those with 'positive family climate', 67% of those with 'intermediate family climate' and 43% of those with 'negative family climate' ($p \ll .04$). Finally, extreme differences were noted between the three groups in relation to the teachers' ratings of 'positive adjustment to deafness.' The children in Group 1 (residential students — deaf parents) were much higher (80%) than those in Groups 2 and 3 respectively (50% and 32%) ($p \ll .001$).

The authors discuss the implication of their findings for the development of intellect and academic achievement; for the development of identity; and for intimacy relationships among adolescents.

A final section of the book presents data from a survey of 516 deaf children in residential schools. Based on teachers' ratings, about 12% of deaf students were judged to be severely emotionally disturbed and a further 19.6% to have milder behavioural problems compared with 2.4% and 7.3% of students in Los Angeles county generally. Characteristics of the disturbed students were found primarily in relation to family situations (intactness, size, age and religion) and some personal characteristics (sex, IQ).

The book is thorough, comprehensive and based on thoughtful and careful studies. It is to be regarded as a pivotal contribution to the literature in this field, comparable in importance to the contributions of Rainer and his colleagues (1963, 1966 and 1970). It goes a step beyond the nature-nurture controversy that characterizes so much of the earlier literature, to look instead at 'the entire life cycle, examining instances of optimal and minimal adjustment and seeking out the antecedents, correlates and consequences of these patterns.'

This is a philosophy complementary to Dinnage (1972) as expressed in her own research summary governing emotional development of the deaf: 'On the whole, evidence about the emotional adjustment of deaf children is drawn from a variety of non-comparable types of investigation which, like all attempted assessments of personality and feeling, implies some confusion about what 'good adjustment' is and whether it can at all easily be measured . . . In any case, it does appear from the research reviewed that the severely and the partially deaf have different patterns of behaviour and that the latter may have both more opportunities and more problems; that differences in parental affection and support affect deaf children as they do any other children, but that deafness, like other handicaps, may make it harder for parents to act with spontaneity and confidence; that emotional deprivation may tend to produce withdrawn, autistic behaviour rather than aggression in both blind and deaf children; and that far more support, guidance, and therapy should be available for these children and their families — although this will not be of value unless the special characteristics and problems of deafness are understood.'

In striking contrast to the prolific literature on psychological problems in deaf and blind children, research into those with *speech* disorder is heavily biased in favour of emotionally based disturbance lacking a clear organic basis. The emphasis undoubtedly reflects the multiplicity of different types of disorder encompassed under this rubric. Apart from such clear-cut examples as disorder secondary to cleft palate, there is the large and composite group with articulation defects, which, in turn, may be subdivided into several separate entities. Another major category of disorder is characterized by complete absence of, or excessive delay in the development of meaningful speech; and finally, there is the group of children who habitually stutter.

While the exact role of psychological factors in each of these conditions has been fiercely debated, the issue is largely limited to the extent and quality of contribution these factors make to the aetiology of the problem. There has been relatively little focus upon emotional consequences as such; and, as in other disorders with a presumed psychosomatic component, the danger of false circular reasoning (based upon cross-sectional studies) is great. Nevertheless, major speech disorder can evoke profound reactions in others, to the extent at times of actually stigmatizing the child, such is the social significance attached to speech. The results previously adduced in respect of clefts is particularly apposite here.

A study by Fitzimmons (1958) using the Children's Apperception Test provides abundant evidence of 'tension-producing symptoms' among children with articulation disorders. The CAT protocols contain frequent references to 'destruction, injury, and mutilation, projection of fear and anxieties, and perceptions of parents in authoritarian, demanding roles.' In general, the 70 children with abnormal speech were more deviant in developmental, psychosocial and educational variables than were the 70 matched controls. What is of interest is that the author interprets these findings as evidence that 'language problems are psychogenic in aetiology.' 'A non-organic speech problem may be satisfying a need for the reduction of internal tension.' Yet, precisely the opposite interpretation could be placed on these same findings — that the symptoms of maladjustment follow from the presence of the basic disorder and its social consequences!

One of the few studies to document objectively the reaction of other children toward those with speech disorders is described by Marge (1966). One hundred and ninety-seven third grade children from a middle class suburban community were studied, using two sociometric questionnaires, a speech rating form and an attitude questionnaire for parents. Thirty-six of the children were judged to have speech difficulties that were moderate or severe; these were compared with a randomly selected control group. The study was carefully executed and the results fairly conclusive, although many of those judged to have speech problems had not been so identified previously by their teachers!

Nevertheless, the results demonstrate clearly that those with speech problems were less popular choices (significantly so) for hypothetical activities involving 'intellectual prowess' and 'social desirability.' (Surprisingly, they were *not* less favoured choices for activities involving speaking skill, *e.g.* someone who would speak for you if you had a sore throat and could not talk!) Of importance is the finding that teachers' responses *also* indicated a preference for normal speaking children, for each of the four activities listed in the sociogramme.

These findings are chiefly of importance in conjunction with the work of Glasner (1949) and Ingram (1959). Both suggest the higher frequency of maladjustment, often requiring psychiatric attention, in children with these disorders. Neither study is conclusive, however, in its results, so that the question must remain open pending greater emphasis on studies designed specifically to separate cause and effect contributions among psychological factors.

C. Cosmetic disorders
Over the years relatively little interest has been displayed in

the psychological consequences of conditions affecting appearance in childhood. Most of the best evidence primarily relates to adults and suggests that the reaction of others to disfigurement may be innate. Four-month-old infants studied by Kagan *et al.* (1966) gave less 'smiling responses' when shown abnormal three-dimensional models of faces than when shown a normal face. In their extensive series of studies using pictures of children with a variety of physical handicaps, Richardson *et al.* (1961) have shown consistently that the visibility of the child's disorder is a salient feature determining the responses of other children. Surprisingly, perhaps, several of Richardson's studies indicate that children with essentially cosmetic disorders, such as obesity, are less preferred than those with orthopaedic disorders (see page 172, Section V). Richardson (1968) states, 'Despite the lack of empirical evidence to support them, associations between personal characteristics and physical appearance continue to exist, perhaps because they serve a number of purposes in the initial social encounter.'

One of the major contributors to this literature is MacGregor. In 1953 she and her colleagues described an extensive psychosocial study of persons with facial deformities receiving plastic surgery. This report is based upon four case histories, one of which deals with a six-year-old child undergoing surgical reconstruction of a congenital malformation of the ear. Despite the relatively minimal nature of the deformity, the detailed case history abundantly reveals the extreme stress imposed on the child and his family by this cosmetic abnormality.

'All his life, Tommy Jonson has lived in an atmosphere that has reflected the values society places on deformity and which his parents and other significant people in his life have absorbed and transmitted to him directly or by implication. At birth he was treated as an atypical infant; his mother was at first not allowed to see him, and a student nurse reported him as 'deformed.'

In summarizing, the authors point out that 'the patient shares the attitudes and prejudices of the society in which he lives.' The contributors all reported marked personality differences between the mildly and severely deformed and comment on the paradoxical manner in which many patients who are 'severely disfigured complained less bitterly than the mildly disfigured.'

In a subsequent conference report, MacGregor (1963) describes the problem of rehabilitating patients with facial disfigurement. And in another very sensitive discussion of psychosocial problems associated with facial deformities, several cases are chosen to illustrate the general principles observed in a study of 115 patients receiving plastic surgery (MacGregor, 1951). One of the patients was a 31-year-old adult who had a birth injury resulting in complete paralysis of the right side of his face. Extensive quotations describe the reactions of his parents, school teachers, and colleagues to illustrate the depth of response displayed by the average person.

Upon entering school he soon learned that something was 'wrong with his face'. 'It was my teachers who first made me self-conscious. They would stop me in the middle of a recitation and ask me what was the matter with my face. They would say, "Try and control it. Don't talk on one side of your mouth like that".' MacGregor continues, 'Tom came home from school everyday and did not linger on the streets with other children who began to taunt him . . . In high school his life was similar — he preferred poor grades to the ridicule and staring of other students. He did not try to make friends nor did he participate in school dances or other social activities.'

In discussing his decision to undergo surgery in the hope of improving the paralysis, Tom says — 'I can't be worse off than I am and even if it fails, if by having the operation I can help someone who comes after me, I'm glad to do it. I'm filled with pent-up emotion; I can't laugh or smile or do anything. I have long periods of depression and resentment. I'm terribly sensitive . . . I've been so handicapped all my life, so ridiculed and humiliated, that anything is worth trying.'

MacGregor emphasizes that 'the patient's feelings of inadequacy and hostility, his periods of depression, are due less to his deformity than to his reactions to the actual and anticipated responses of others toward his appearance. We see here the influential role the group may play in determining the kind of interpretation an individual places upon his own deformity. Called derogatory nicknames by his contemporaries, offered jobs where he would have a minimum of social contact, and characterized as being "tough", seemed to accentuate behaviour patterns of negative nature.'

It is from a similar clinical base that Easson (1966) describes parental reactions to facial deformity in young infants. Likewise the reports by Berk (1963) on the psychological significance of contact lenses on children and youths, and by Bryt (1966) on candidates for plastic surgery. In contrast, Schoenfeld (1964) employed both the Rorschach and the TAT to elicit the nature of body-image disturbances in adolescents with 'inappropriate sexual development' resulting from underlying medical disorders.

Although such abnormalities may not properly be regarded as 'cosmetic' in the strict sense, they undoubtedly represent a highly sensitive manifestation of concern with bodily appearance. The details of the test results are not given but the author is emphatic in asserting the importance of body-image as a factor in determining adolescent adjustment.

Based on his review of more than 600 adolescents with sexually inappropriate development, Schoenfeld is convinced that disturbed body-image results in deviant behaviour and maladaptation. He claims that parental over-solicitude and emotional conflicts in early childhood exaggerate the reactions of individuals, and recommends that treatment be directed toward 'restructuring the body-image.' Although a number of divergent diagnostic groups were included, *e.g.* breast abnormalities, eunuchoidism, delayed puberty and dwarfism, Schoenfeld concludes that factors of importance 'common to all groups is the age of onset of the defect and the personality adjustment made prior to its appearance.' These together 'wielded considerable influence on the basic mechanisms producing the body-image.'

Although relatively rare, a related condition of similar and equally major psychological import is extrophy of the bladder. Feinberg *et al.* (1974) record that about 200 children with extrophy and complete epispadias are born each year in the U.S. Although new surgical techniques are available for dealing with some aspects of this severe congenital anomaly, concern about urinary and sexual function create major adjustment difficulties. 'While our surgical results have been good, our thinking and that of the parents has been so taken up with the technical aspects of getting the children to heal, that we have often failed to give them all the psychological support they need.'

To assess their adjustment difficulties, 14 children were interviewed along with their parents. Two major problems were identified — embarrassment due to wetness and odour resulting from incontinence, and concern about the appearance of the genitalia. Marked improvements were noted following surgery but, nonetheless, teasing, anxiety, and difficulties in sexual adaptation persisted. A wide variety of areas warranting information and counselling are identified, and the authors suggest the need for an 'ongoing guidance team which becomes involved with the family at the birth of the infant . . . and which extends its services into young adulthood . . . to help children gain understanding, to enable them to ventilate feelings and fantasies and resolve conflicts.'

Another major area of cosmetic abnormality is the scarring resulting from burns. Vigliano, Hart and Singer (1964) studied 10 children long after recovery and discovered 'lasting emotional maladjustments in both the children and their mothers, related at least in part to the trauma of the burn.' Several projective techniques were employed to help the respondents express their feelings (Holtzman inkblot, CAT, Symonds Picture Story Test), and the mothers were interviewed in detail by a psychiatrist and social worker. The small size of the group is recognized as a limitation but in the investigators' opinion the evidence of adjustment problems in most cases is of sufficient magnitude 'to justify, in ordinary clinical practice, treatment in an outpatient child psychiatric clinic.' The authors also speculate on possibilities for preventing emotional problems through 'bedside interpretations' that might contribute to preserving a relatively stable body-image and reducing anxiety over the vulnerability of the body. The potential value of discussion groups for the mothers is also raised in view of the fact that nine of the children and eight of the mothers were judged to be seriously disturbed.

Scoliosis is a relatively common condition affecting

appearance, and is particularly distressing when, as so often, it occurs among adolescent girls. Using the Holtzman inkblot technique, Draw-a-Person Test, and a sentence completion procedure, Myers and her colleagues (1970) found evidence of poor adjustment in nine of 25 girls studied. In view of the fact that six of the nine had been referred because of behavioural problems, the results cannot be generalized, but the observations about coping behaviour are of interest. The use of intrapsychic defence mechanisms, such as identification, denial, intellectualization, reaction formation and displacement are discussed, as is the use of motor activity to help cope with the stresses imposed.

An 'initial storm' of psychological upheaval was usually followed by a period of fairly normal daily activities except in a few cases. In those coping well, understanding of the illness and the reason for the bracing procedure used, the role of family support and encouragement, an optimistic view of outcome with a definite termination time, and the support and interest of the medical staff — each played an important role. The age of onset also appears to be of importance: in agreement with other investigators, the authors feel the girls were helped by the long period of normality before the onset of their condition.

The most common and obvious 'cosmetic' abnormality involves major deviations in stature. Although some work relates excessive height to abnormal behaviour, particularly antisocial behaviour, most of this is based upon boys with chromosomal disorders. It is therefore reasoned that the behavioural disturbances have a 'genetic' rather than psychologic basis (Hook and Kim, 1971). More commonly, interest has focused upon the consequences of dwarfism, whether due to normal variations in growth or endocrine disorder. Generally speaking, most people, including parents, tend to treat a child of excessively short stature in accordance with his apparent age, i.e. as a much younger child. The children, in turn, respond as would younger children, which, as in the case of scholastic under-achievement, may explain many of the behavioural consequences they experience.

Money and Pollitt (1966) studied 17 dwarfs who had been treated with human growth hormone. Through interviews and structured observations they demonstrated that 'the degree of psychomaturation achieved tended to parallel the degree to which the dwarf had been treated socially according to age and not size.' In only five of the children was maturation judged to be 'adequate' and many of those whose maturation was 'distorted' or 'deficient' were found to employ a variety of psychodynamic mechanisms ranging from elective mutism to school phobia to cope with their distress.

Although in many instances growth hormone treatment was medically successful, the responses of the patients to their increased growth was often ambivalent or even antagonistic. The authors caution that particularly in the case of chronic disability to which the subject has become attuned, patients may not place the same value on therapeutic outcome as do their physicians. The demands of what they term 'the readjustment syndrome' are frequently taxing and may even result in a desire to discontinue treatment. Unlike other disorders, the psychological responses to dwarfism tend to be fairly uniform: 'A dwarf tends to manifest personality mechanisms of retreat that belong in the general category of dissociation, denial and inhibition . . . There does not seem to be much place in the psychology of dwarfism for personality mechanisms that pertain to aggressive and destructive mastery.'

In view of the pervasive importance of body-image in the development of self-concept, there are surprisingly few studies of maladjustment in relation to dermatological conditions such as severe acne, psoriasis, or eczema. One exception is the report by Bender and Faretra (1963) describing the psychological reactions to depigmentation in a 14-year-old Negro girl. 'She felt deformed, inadequate, and ugly, though she was otherwise a pretty, well-developed girl. She was happiest at home, where her appearance was accepted and rarely mentioned, but she became hostile and aggressive if attention were drawn to her skin . . .'

The authors conclude, 'Body-image disturbances undoubtedly occur in every illness or abnormality. The severity and prognosis of psychological disturbance to physical illness depend much on the attitudes and management of the child's problems by persons caring for him.'

The categorization of chronic disorders into five major groups, according to type of disability, is clearly arbitrary. There are many conditions that do not fit well in any category and others, such as cleft lip-palate, that could be placed in more than one group. Most children with clefts have difficulty with speech but this is not, properly speaking, an example of a 'special sense' disorder. Clefts often produce a slight degree of cosmetic disfigurement even after repair, and only on a case-by-case basis could it be decided which aspect was the more salient psychologically. We discuss here some of the research undertaken on the consequences of these conditions, primarily because the speech abnormality may also be viewed as having 'cosmetic' significance in the broad sense of the term.

Spierstersbach (1973) conducted an extensive study of the psychosocial aspects of cleft palate in an attempt to relate the nature and severity of adjustment problems to the adequacy of the information parents were given, to parental attitudes and patterns of response, and to the management procedures used by those caring for these children. The study involved 175 children with cleft lip, palate or both, and their parents, and a matched sample of 175 controls. The procedure included detailed interviews, medical examinations, psychological testing with the WISC and the Vineland, and several speech and hearing tests.

The absence of detailed cross-tabulations and statistical tests prevents definitive conclusions from being drawn. Nevertheless, the evidence *in toto* suggests that a majority of the children studied were maladjusted in one way or another and that many of their parents received grossly inadequate information, advice, counselling and support from the professional personnel with whom they had come in contact. Spierstersbach first makes a plea for more study of the course of 'accommodation' to conditions of this nature, but, based on the interview data, he also advocates, vociferously, the need for more counselling at each successive state of the illness and its treatment. He adds that 'parents of children with clefts are frequently naive observers' and suggests that more time be devoted to helping parents become a more effective part of the habilitation team. Because of the potential for 'complete habilitation' through surgery, he notes that there is a danger in overstating the case for 'normality.' Rather the population of children with this disorder should be recognized as a heterogeneous one, further efforts being needed to identify factors that make some children maladjusted while others, often with more severe abnormalities, cope well.

In an earlier section we describe some of the findings of Smith and McWilliams (1966, 1968) that suggest that these children are 'less creative than noncleft children in certain verbal and nonverbal areas' and that they frequently have specific psycholinguistic disabilities that may handicap them in their scholastic achievement. Although the latter may be viewed as a fairly direct consequence of the organic disorder, it is likely that in both cases, 'certain psychosocial variables . . . mediate between the physical disability and the child's behaviour.' Again the role of the home is emphasized, particularly those situations in which the habilitation process itself may limit opportunities for self-fulfilment.

This view is partially supported by the findings of Clifford (1969). His study was based on the assumption that 'selective aspects of the environment acquire subjective . . . meanings as a function of previous experiences . . . such as the onset of a symptom (or clinical entity).' Clifford compared the meaning of the symptoms associated with cleft palate with those associated with asthma, using the semantic differential technique; a series of self-report questions to assess the current impact of the symptom directly; another series to assess changes that might occur with symptom loss; and a fourth to assess perceptions of parental acceptance at birth. The current impact ratings showed no significant differences between any of the groups (palate only, lip and palate, total lip-palate, and asthmatics). Of interest is that 'palate only' patients perceived a higher degree of acceptance by parents than did those with both cleft lip and palate, and asthmatics were significantly higher than either of the cleft groups. None of the self-concept measures using the sematic differential showed significant differences.

We interpret the results of this study to indicate the salience of the cosmetic component of the lip-palate combination as well as emphasizing the importance of age of onset of a child's chronic condition.

D. Locomotor disorders

The conditions described under this heading have only one thing in common — their restrictive effect on the child's ability to move about freely, due to lesions of the muscular or skeletal systems. Of course, locomotion may equally be restricted as a consequence of CNS damage, but because this so often involves other disabilities, we have dealt with it separately. The same applies to severe involvement of the cardiovascular or pulmonary systems, both of which may affect locomotion indirectly; and strictly speaking, rheumatoid arthritis should also be included with locomotor disorders, but because of the controversy surrounding its possible psychosomatic origins, it too has been allotted separate consideration.

What remains are those disorders generally classified as 'physical handicaps' although, as indicated previously (page 22, Section I) this term is especially misleading. Even the designation 'orthopaedic' is not sufficiently inclusive, although it probably comes closest to the most acceptable and commonly adopted clinical diagnostic rubric. The psychological importance of these disorders lies primarily in the effects that restricted mobility may have in curtailing achievement of important goals or even routine daily activities. This view is derived from field theory previously described under the heading of somato-psychology (see page 24). For Adlerians, the problem may be viewed as one of 'organ inferiority' whereas for Freudians, it is seen largely in terms of body-image perception and self-concept. Our concern is less with constructing a theoretical substrate for the relationship between locomotor disorders and adjustment, as with examining the evidence empirically in the hope of deriving a pragmatic model from which prevention or therapeutic intervention may evolve.

Barker *et al.* (1953) reviewed more than 100 papers dealing with the 'somato-psychological significance of crippling,' placing heavy emphasis on the importance of attitudes — attitudes of parents, society in general, and of course, of the 'crippled' person himself. Cruickshank, too, although including cerebral palsy, thoroughly reviewed the earlier literature on psychological aspects of crippled children (1963).

In the second volume of the review by Dinnage (1972), her section on 'locomotor' handicaps deals exclusively with spina bifida and the thalidomide syndrome. These examples are quoted to illustrate the problem of properly defining this category of handicap; in this sense, including conditions such as poliomyelitis is open to debate.

From an historical point of view, one of the earliest studies to employ both objective measures of adjustment and a group of controls is that of Gates (1946). Only 18 subjects were included, most of whom had an orthopaedic disorder (with the exception of one child with heart disease). The controls were drawn from both siblings and unrelated healthy children of similar background. A battery of tests (most of which are no longer in use) were employed and, in addition, each child wrote a brief autobiographical account of incidents felt to be important in influencing their opinions, etc. In brief, the results showed no statistically significant differences for any of the objective measures, although the scores of the disabled were generally lower than those of the controls.

Another study of historical importance is that of Mussen and Newman (1958). It begins by recognizing that some previous inconsistencies in attempting to relate handicap to maladjustment may be explained by the relative insensitivity of standardized pencil and paper tests compared with the greater yield of less structured procedures. They point to the findings of Broida et al. (1950) and Cruickshank (1952) as demonstrating significant difficulties in interpersonal relations and greater immaturity among the disabled. More importantly, however, Mussen and Newman recognize the danger of examining group differences alone, which prompted them to examine some of the antecedent factors more closely. They were influenced by the arguments of Dembo and her colleagues (1948) that 'the adjustment process called acceptance of loss was found to permit the disabled person to face his disability without devaluating himself.' Their concept of 'acceptance' and its central importance will be elaborated further in Section V (page 181). Here, it is of relevance chiefly in understanding Mussen and Newman's hypothesis that strong dependency needs characterize the well-adjusted handicapped whereas strong achievement needs are more prevalent among the poorly adjusted.

Teacher's ratings were used to assess personality characteristics presumed to be related to adjustment; TAT tests to assess achievement and dependency needs. The results clearly support the hypothesis, and help to clarify the psychological significance of the acceptance of loss in determining the child's adjustment. Acceptance in this context implies the development of a system of needs compatible with the disability, and in turn, acknowledgement of dependency within limits (see page 181, Section V). At the same time, the authors emphasize that acceptance of dependency is not incompatible with the desire for independence or self-assertion.

In more recent years many of these basic findings have been replicated by other investigators using quite different approaches and techniques. For example, Downing et al. (1961) used a semantic differential test to assess the concept of self-evaluation. Forty-one children ranging in age from seven to 19, and hospitalized for immobilization, during some two years, for the treatment of Legg-Perthes disease, were given the test following discharge from hospital. The results convey little about the extent of self-devaluation, but do confirm the reliability of the procedure and demonstrate its range of potential applications.

A more traditional approach was adopted by McFie and Robertson (1973) in their study of children with thalidomide deformities. Apart from the data on intelligence test scores referred to previously (p.103), results were obtained from the Vineland Social Maturity Scale. These indicated that although performance was generally related to degree of handicap, many inconsistencies were found, which suggested that 'the attitudes of the parents and the personalities of the children themselves were important additional factors.' Based on the children's behaviour during testing, and separating from their parents, assessments were also made of emotional adjustment. On the whole, emotional adjustment appeared 'fairly good,' though it was observed that 'there were fewer anxious or depressed children and more who were cheerful and self-confident among those with the more extensive malformations.' (Kellmer-Pringle and Fiddes (1970) also noted that the least deformed appeared to be most aware of their deficiency — a further reference to marginality — see pages 118 and 171.)

Another example of the traditional approach to assessment of body-image is provided by Wysocki and Whitney (1965). Most of the 50 'crippled' children in their study did, indeed have an orthopaedic disorder, although 13 had polio and eight, cerebral palsy. The results of the Draw-a-Person test were compared with 50 healthy children of similar age and IQ distribution. Of the 15 aspects of the drawings that were compared, eight showed statistically significant differences, with the disabled children more often drawing larger heads, figures of the opposite sex, large figure size, unusual placement, shading, etc. The technique is of interest but unless unsubstantiated assumptions about the meaning of their findings are to be accepted uncritically, they tell us little about the adjustment of these children beyond the fact that they may have a different image of their bodies.

Two studies of children with osteogenesis imperfecta are of special interest because they both suggest that these children, in spite of multiple fractures, severe deformities, and growth disturbances that often result in dwarfism, appear to be unusually well-adjusted. In an attempt to survey all cases of this disorder in Sweden, Smars and Berfenstram (1961) succeeded in identifying 190 patients who were investigated by interview and examination. At the time of the study, the patients ranged in age from one to 29 years. No specific information is provided about psychological adjustment directly, but based on an array of indirect indices (school performance, vocational achievements, independent living, marriage, etc.), the authors note that 'even patients with very serious functional reduction often had an amazing ability for adaptation.' They go on to speculate about the possibility that these subjects may have special intellectual or other qualities that have enabled them to achieve this high level of adaptation. Some evidence that the group were, in fact, exceptionally intelligent, is offered, as well as a consistent finding of 'positive attitude, optimism, and drive.' The authors conclude, 'The general mental state of the patient, his psychological balance and attitude to his own situation, and not least his intellectual capacity, seem to be more important factors (in achieving adaptation) than the reduction of physical function.'

In view of the reliance on 'indirect' measures in the Swedish study, it might be tempting to discount these conclusions or attribute them to a 'halo effect,' based on the expectations of the investigators. However, a more recent report by Reite *et al.* (1972) replicates and expands the earlier observations. Although incomplete at the time they were reported, these findings appeared promptly because the authors were intrigued by the relatively normal emotional and cognitive development they observed. Twelve children were studied, each severely incapacitated and disfigured by osteogenesis imperfecta. Their ages were between six and 17 at the time of the study and ten were markedly deformed, dwarfed and confined to a wheelchair. The evaluation included a psychiatric interview with parents and child, an intelligence test, and the Draw-a-Person test.

The authors reported that 'as a group, our youngsters were remarkably well-adjusted, pleasant and at ease with others. They had never been behaviour problems and none exhibited overt psychopathology, nor did they have related complaints. All had average or better school performance, although the educational mode varied from home tutoring to regular classroom attendance.' They also noted that children who had been allowed maximum freedom in personal activity, despite the inherent dangers, exhibited the least severe distortion of body-image on the DAP (*cf* the findings of Mattsson and others in relation to children with haemophilia).

In speculating on the reason for these unexpected findings, the intriguing suggestion is submitted that an increase in rate of cellular oxidation (a component of the basic metabolic process in this disorder) may favourably influence the central nervous system generally, and cognitive maturational patterns in particular. In support of this view, cyclic AMP activity has been linked with the regulation or modulation of affective behaviour, and, in turn, OI has been linked with cyclic AMP. Thus the fact that these children are 'uniformly noted . . . to be cheerful and not prone to mood swings or depressed periods,' may be related to the higher affective tone resulting from this biochemical relationship. It is suggested that 'such a persistent mild euphoria could serve a protective function against other illness-related ego dystonic forces.'

One of the fundamental problems facing the group of children with locomotor disorders is that they often experience prolonged periods of immobilization due to treatment. Some, in addition, have their activities severely restricted to protect them from harm, or simply because they are unable to engage in pursuits requiring mobility of the limbs. Although analytically oriented investigators (*e.g.* Anna Freud and Mittelman) have claimed that sustained restrictions in mobility during early developmental stages may have significant effects on subsequent behaviour, these last two studies suggest that this is by no means invariable.

In a further attempt to isolate a 'pure strain' of locomotor disability (and so avoid the confusion which results from including heterogeneous disorders within this broad category), Siller (1960) studied only those children who had had limb amputations. The subjects in his investigation were 52 children between two and 17 years of age; about half had amputations of the upper extremity, the other half of the lower. (Ten also had other anomalies.) Each child, plus the majority of the parents, was interviewed by a psychologist using a semi-structured format; in addition, a battery of projective and objective measures was employed. The data were analysed to yield information about reactions to disability, parental acceptance, social sensitivity and general adjustment. The case reports from which these variables were assessed were rated independently by three psychologists; the agreement was generally high.

The most frequent reactions to the disability were denial coupled with various compensatory mechanisms such as independent strivings to 'reconstitute their feelings of self-esteem and sense of personal worthiness.' In spite of these defenses, 40% were judged to be disturbed or to display 'inadequate adjustment.' There was a non-significant relationship between adjustment and parental acceptance which, in 63% of cases, was rated as 'average or above average.' The relationship between social sensitivity and maladjustment (as might be expected) was highly significant, and somewhat related to parental acceptance. Although few important associations could be traced between aetiology of the amputation and the psychosocial measures, in the main, those with congenital amputations fared best, particularly with respect to overall adjustment.

A concept introduced by Siller to help explain some of these findings, is that of a 'restitution-avoidance dichotomy'; an attempt to categorize specific reactions to disability in terms of their common function. It is suggested that the child's primary mode of responding to the amputation is (a) to attempt restitution for the loss and (b) to avoid the implications of the loss. A third possible category,. designated 'insecurity reactions,' includes inferiority feelings, shame, fearfulness, and dependency. These categories of reaction were found to be related to sensitivity, acceptance and adjustment, thereby pointing to both their pragmatic usefulness and theoretical validity, even though they were derived *post-hoc,* and hence must be viewed at teleological.

Much of the remaining literature in this area tackles the question of frequency of maladjustment in locomotor disorder through studies of less well-defined groups, often using subjective rather than objective measures. For example, McMichael's (1971) account of a group of physically handicapped children and their families deals with fifty children who were pupils in a special primary school in London. Her main sources of information were derived from a standard interview questionnaire which she herself administered, and a teacher's questionnaire based on that used in the National Survey of Health and Development. The shortcomings of this method are apparent — the sample is relatively small, mixed and unrepresentative; and the information, largely 'clinical.' (However, five of the interviews were repeated independently and the results compared; and other sources of school information were included.)

This study is complementary to those described earlier. As Tizard states in the preface: 'There is an intimacy about case studies which is invariably lacking in studies of larger samples . . . For a case study such as this . . . a "control" group would serve little purpose; and even to know the comparative frequency of various problems is perhaps of less importance than is the knowledge that for the families studied medical, educational, social and material problems occur in all their complexity in a high proportion of cases.'

About one-half of the children studied had disorders of the CNS—including eight with the residua of polio. Bearing this in mind the referral rate for child guidance of 24%, while high, is not surprising, even though it is about three times the average from ordinary schools. The actual problems ranged from anxiety, withdrawal, tantrums and aggression to enuresis and sexual precocity. No single pattern predominated, other than elements of anxiety. Using a measure of maladjustment based on interview responses independently obtained from mothers and teachers, 56% were rated as having moderate to severe emotional difficulties. The author also records a high rate of parental rejection (31%), severe degrees of anxiety and over-projection (56%), and 'considerable difficulties in adjusting to the handicap' in 21% of the siblings.

A similar British study on a larger scale are the composite reports to the Carnegie United Kingdom Trust dealing with the problems of 600 'handicapped' children and their families (1964). About 200 children were studied in each of two cities — Glasgow and Sheffield, and in a rural area in the West Midland counties. Although a wide variety of 'handicapping disorders' were included, e.g. vision, speech, hearing, cerebral palsy, etc., each area included at least one group with orthopaedic conditions or those classified as 'physically handicapped.' In many respects this is an exemplary study — not as a scientific investigation, but in terms of its comprehensiveness and detailed consideration of the child in the context of his community. It is one of the few studies which emphasizes that what may represent problems for children or their parents in large urban communities, may be no trouble for those in rural areas — and vice versa. Reflecting this important 'parochial' bias, each of the three study groups proceeded independently, some using more quantifiable methods than others. It is therefore, difficult to tease out figures relating separately to emotional adjustment in locomotor disorders, but the general impression is that at least one-third of the children in this group had emotional difficulties added to their physical disabilities.

One value of this and a subsequent report — *Living With Handicap* (Younghusband et al. 1970) by a working party on children with 'special needs' — is the emphasis placed on the mundane, everyday problems that contribute so greatly to the burden on parents and hence to the adjustment of their children. 'I imagine that the greatest cross the parent of a handicapped child has to bear is exhaustion' writes Anne Allen in the appendix. Although in neither report are emotional problems as such dominant, they are abundantly reflected in the needs expressed and in the recommendations made.

Asked to indicate their personal and social needs, parents listed relief from full-time care, financial hardship, social isolation, inferiority and guilt feelings, attitudes of neighbours, lack of advice and information, transportation, housing and equipment. In both reports the lack of co-ordination of existing services and the need for new services stands out clearly (see page 208, Section V).

The specific recommendations in the report to the Carnegie Trust are: (1) Establishment of a co-ordinating agency for diagnosis and action arising therefrom; (2) Establishment of a counselling service; (3) Service in the home; (4) Training of counsellors and workers in the home; (5) Service after-care; (6) Co-ordination of and guidance to home teachers; and (7) Relief to parents. Undoubtedly much more can be done for these children.

The importance of peer-group attitudes also emerged in the study by Centers and Centers (1963a). Using modified sociometric techniques, they found that in classrooms where some of the children had arm amputations, their peers more frequently expressed rejecting attitudes toward them than to other 'able-bodied' children. Another report dealing with the same group of 26 amputees (Centers and Centers, 1963b), describes the results of judges' ratings of the figure drawings of these children, compared with those of 26 matched controls. Although few differences were found, it is of interest that those that were consisted mainly of abnormalities in the drawings of the arms. However, there was little indication of maladjustment as such from the drawings.

Similar findings are reported by Force (1956). A near-sociometric instrument was used to determine the choices of friends, playmates, and workmates in 14 elementary school classes which included 63 physically handicapped children and 360 non-handicapped. As predicted, the handicapped received significantly less choices in each of the three categories. Both groups tended to choose within 'their own groups,' the obvious nature of a child's disability being a factor which influenced the choice in many instances.

A more important, more direct approach to the question of self-image in children with orthopaedic disorder (including a few with cerebral palsy, postpolio, cardiac conditions and diabetes), is found in a study by Richardson *et al.* (1964). The subjects included 107 physically handicapped children aged 9-11 years, compared with 128 non-handicapped children, all of whom were attending a summer camp. An exploratory study yielded 69 empirically-derived content categories, applied in the analysis of self-description and description of others, obtained by interviewing the children. The results suggest that self-descriptions by the handicapped are realistic — they displayed feelings of inability to live up to expectations because of the high values placed by society on physical activities. Some interesting differences emerged between boys and girls; the boys were more concerned about aggression and competition, and often used humour to gain acceptance.

The issues underlying the process of socialization in young, severely handicapped children have been reviewed by Battle (1974). She raises the important question of whether there are, in fact, 'critical periods' for acquiring socialization skills, and whether the effects of early deprivation, so common among these children, can be reversed. Battle emphasizes that as the child grows older he drops further and further behind his normal peers; she cogitates about the long-term effects of such disruptions. These themes are echoed by Poznanski (1973), whose emphasis is primarily on the feelings of the parents, and by Bentovim (1972a, b), who deals both with the parents' attitudes toward the handicapped pre-school child, and the effect on that child's early emotional development. Both papers, however, deal with handicap rather globally so that the specific effects on locomotor disorder as such are not sufficiently isolated to warrant further comment.

E. Systemic disorders

1. *Diabetes*

Firm conclusions about the psychosocial consequences of juvenile diabetes are difficult to reach because of the very close connection between emotional factors and neurohumoural functioning. One major stream of investigation continues to explore the possible role of psychological factors in aetiology — such studies, for example, as Stein and Charles, 1971 or Geiger *et al.* 1973 — which seek to establish that diabetes is a consequence of psychological stress in a physiologically susceptible individual.

The Hungarian team (Geiger and his co-workers) studied 58 diabetic children using detailed histories and projective tests in an attempt to determine retrospectively the significance of various neurotic symptoms. Forty-seven per cent of the children were found to be depressed and the investigators assert that in all but six cases symptoms were present *before* the onset of the illness.

The study by Stein and Charles encompassed 76 patients with an average age of 18 years and a control group with other chronic illnesses matched by age, social class, sex, race and religion. Sixty-nine per cent of the diabetics compared with 19% of the controls, had suffered parental loss or severe family disturbance, and in 77% of the diabetics the losses occurred *before* the illness was diagnosed.

The significance of these findings is open to question. They must be examined alongside extensive evidence suggesting that emotional disturbance found among diabetics is primarily a *result* of the illness and not an antecedent. Both Sterky (1963) and Swift *et al.* (1967) have studied this aspect of the question using reasonably representative samples and carefully selected control groups.

Sterky's survey of 145 cases comprised the majority of juvenile diabetics of school age traceable in Stockholm at the time of the study. These cases were paired with non-diabetics of similar sex, age, grade and social class, and although the total frequency of 'mentally disturbed' subjects was the same in both groups, the diabetics showed several symptoms much more frequently than their healthy peers. In particular 'emotional lability,' 'aggression' and 'difficulties with companions' were more frequently found among the diabetics, especially among the girls. When those with emotional disturbance were compared with symptom-free subjects, two significant differences were found: the disturbed children had an increased frequency of mentally disturbed mothers; they were also more often judged to be in 'poor' diabetic control. Of interest, moreover, is that Sterky found a tendency in the diabetics both toward an increase in cases with symptoms with advancing age, and an increase in mental symptoms per case, whereas the reverse held true for the controls.

In their comprehensive study of 50 juvenile diabetics and 50 individually matched healthy controls, Swift, Seidman and Stein (1967) hypothesized that children with diabetes would show more emotional disturbance and social maladjustment; that their parents would differ from parents of controls in child-rearing patterns and emotional relationships; and that poorly controlled diabetics would be more disturbed than those who were well-controlled. Using a large battery of projective and objective tests, interviews and psychiatric evaluations, each of these hypotheses was supported. Diabetics were 'more abnormal than the non-diabetic controls in psychiatric classification, more extreme in dependence-independence balance, less adequate in self-percept, had greater manifest and latent anxiety, more pathological sexual identification, greater constriction, more pathological hostility and greater oral preoccupation.' (Each of these differences was statistically significant when compared with the controls.)

In addition it was reported that the emotional tone of the home was poorer for the diabetics, and both mother's and father's relationships with the children were more often deviant in one direction or another, *e.g.* maternal protection or neglect. The major variables related to level of control were home adjustment ratings, psychiatric classification, self-perception, and dependence-independence.

These are undoubtedly two of the better studies culled from the conflicting literature on adjustment in juvenile diabetes. The findings accord with those of Zeidel (1970) and Barcai (1970), as well as with the general conclusions reached by

Treuting (1962), based on his extensive review of the literature. They conflict, however, with many of the older, uncontrolled and less systematic reports.

Studies such as Swift's emphasize the importance of home circumstances in facilitating the child's ability to cope with the stresses imposed by an illness such as diabetes. The relationship between successful coping, defined in psychological terms, and level of control achieved, is not however clear-cut. For example, Tietz and Vidmar (1972) and Koski (1969) both fail to identify any consistent pattern of relationships between diabetic control and such illness variables as age of onset or duration, or with family variables such as degree of intactness, psychopathology or knowledge about diabetes. The American study isolates the importance of family psychopathology, whereas the Finnish report stresses both illness variables and internal and external coping processes in relation to the level of control achieved.

In view of the heavy emphasis placed on the need to instruct the juvenile diabetic and his parents in details of the illness and its management, it is surprising that so few studies have demonstrated convincing links beteen level of understanding and level of control. Studies generally reveal that the level of knowledge shown by children and their parents is highly correlated (*e.g.* Collier *et al.* 1971) but that it falls far short of what most physicians would like (Etzwiler, 1962). Summer camp experience appears to increase knowledge significantly, according to Karp *et al.* (1970); while Weill and Sussman (1961) offer some evidence to show that it also influences the child's adjustment favourably, which in turn results in rather better diabetic control.

2. *Haemophilia*

Pilling (1973), in her annotated bibliography of children with chronic medical problems, noted with respect to research on haemophilia that there were 'no studies in which proper controls were included, from which comparisons with the emotional adjustment of these children could be made.' Attention is called to the studies of Mattsson and his colleagues (1966, 1971), Spencer and Behar (1969) and Agle (1964), each of which found relatively low rates of psychiatric disorder but a strong association between maladjustment and parental relationships.

Mattsson's initial study was of 35 children. Based on interviews and observations, he concluded that 'the majority of patients and their parents showed a good adaptation to the illness. The mothers, in particular, played an essential role in promoting a healthy personality development.' Mattsson notes that 'In addition to the use of reasonable motor activities and compensatory intellectual pursuits, the patients employed some common psychic defenses to support the adaptive process,' *e.g.* denial, isolation of feelings, intellectualization, identification. (These findings contrast with the work of Browne *et al.* (1960) in which many of the 28 patients studied were 'outwardly docile, passive, often appearing depressed, but subtly rebellious'; and this inhibited pattern was related in all but one case to the mother's excessive anxiety.) In Mattsson's group the few children who were poorly adjusted had either 'acquiesced to the mother's overprotection and led restricted lives, or they had rebelled . . . and showed recurrent risk-taking behaviour.'

One intriguing line of investigation, analagous to the efforts to link diabetic control with psychological states, is the attempt to explore potential associations between emotional stress and spontaneous bleeding in haemophilia (see page 175, Section V). Agle (1964) studied 16 adults with this disorder using non-directive interviews. Psychiatric syndromes, *e.g.* anxiety states and recurrent depression, were found in eight; phobic states in four; nine patients displayed recurrent risk-taking behaviour; ten patients reported 'multiple episodes of apparently spontaneous bleeding that have followed a situation that has been emotionally stressful to them or when they have anticipated such a situation.' Although this evidence is far from objective, it is of interest that eight patients noted an improvement in their clinical state following a change in behaviour from passive dependence to more independence; this impression was substantiated in five cases by reduction in hospitalizations, transfusions, etc.

Further evidence for the close relationship between psyche and soma in this disorder comes from the work of Garlinghouse and Sharp (1968). They studied 18 children with haemophilia, most of whom were between nine and 14 years, using the Colvin Silhouette Test to obtain an estimate of self-concept. A measure of stress (the Schedule of Recent Experience Questionnaire) was used alongside a record of bleeding episodes to examine interrelations between these variables. The group as a whole had a high mean self-concept score. The only significant correlations found were between reported stress and bleeding episodes ($p \ll .05$), although there was a tendency for these to decrease with increasing levels of self-perception. When bleeding episodes as a source of stress were removed from the stress score, however, the correlations between stress and bleeding were markedly reduced. The authors conclude, 'In view of the fact that the self-concept acts as a mediator between the environment and the perception of stress by the self, the findings . . . give some evidence that the self-concept of the haemophilic child may afford some protection against the spontaneous bleeding episodes within a certain threshold of stress.'

Olch (1971b) compared Rorschach reponses, need for achievement scores and figure drawings with normative data available for these measures, using a sample of 45 haemophiliacs aged two to 21 years. While commenting that 'the remarkable resemblance noted among haemophiliacs, diabetics and asthmatics does indeed suggest that central aspects of personality development are affected and extreme forms of adaptation are evoked among those who suffer a chronic, serious physical disorder,' the author cautions, 'Nevertheless, an impressive aspect of this study was that a single, typical haemophilic personality was not isolated. Personal reaction styles overshadowed group patterns . . . Diverse psychological strengths as well as disabling features were manifested. Where maladjustment was apparent, this was the result of many factors and could not be attributed solely to the physical condition.'

Olch's findings emphasize the importance of age at the time of psychological assessment. She found that the five to seven-year-olds had a high degree of anxiety, intense feelings of inadequacy and social uneasiness. Those eight to 12-years of age were essentially passive and lacking in spontaneity and 'keenly aware that they differed physically from others.' In contrast, the young adolescents were active, resistant and independent; many exhibited negativism and risk-taking attitudes, whereas the oldest boys showed the greatest personality constriction.

A more recent study by Salk, Hilgartner and Granich (1972), while emphasizing the relatively good adjustment made by the majority of children and their families studied (n = 26), also illustrates the many ways in which family life is disrupted and stressed by a child with a severe chronic illness. A series of highly specific suggestions are offered for enhancing adjustment and reducing family impact, emphasizing in particular the need for guidance and counselling services, group meetings, and educational materials. Several of these suggestions were actually put into practice with a group of young haemophiliacs hospitalized for research purposes over an extended period (Dowling, 1960), in an effort to counteract dependency patterns.

3. *Cystic fibrosis*
Within the large and distinctive body of literature dealing with the dying child, children with cystic fibrosis occupied until recently a tragically large place. In the past decade, however, the prognosis for this disorder has greatly improved with many more children now surviving into adulthood. Accordingly the quality of life and in particular the emotional stability of children obliged to live under covert threat of death, is of special import. Indeed, those who care for them have recently come to realize that the energies previously devoted to insuring their survival must now be directed to insuring that psychosocial problems do not undermine what has been accomplished.

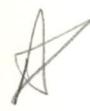

This 'agonizing reappraisal' is best reflected in a recent book edited by Patterson, Denning and Kutscher (1973). Their approach is essentially clinical; for the most part preoccupied with the issue of death and dying. There is, to be sure, a vague awareness that these children need help, guidance and counselling, as do their families, but little evidence that it is being systematically provided in most of the centres. Farkas and Schnell, for example, describe in their section (pp. 202-209) a proposal to study family adjustment, which includes a two-hour battery of psychological tests to measure anxiety, guilt, depression, adjustment and time perspective, but unfortunately no data are presented.

In contrast, Gayton and Friedman (1973) have reviewed seven papers in which actual data on the psychosocial consequences of CF has been assembled. Even here, however, the emphasis is more upon the plight of families than the distress of the children themselves. As the authors point out, although several papers report 'considerable emotional upset in the child with cystic fibrosis' it is impossible to obtain accurate figures on the prevalence of psychological or social maladjustment because of the manner in which the studies were designed. 'Most of the studies, for example, utilized either clinical impressions obtained from psychiatric interviews or test data obtained from abbreviated projective techniques . . .' Nor do any of the studies include normal controls, so that conclusions are obviously limited.

4. *Asthma*
As with several other specific disorders, the psychosocial aspects of asthma remain the subject of controversy. The debate centres upon the same basic questions raised by King (1955) in relation to rheumatoid arthritis: 1) Do the majority of these patients evidence some common and typical personality and psychosocial characteristics? 2) If so, are they specific to the disorder? 3) If they are specific, are they premorbid traits or secondary to the disease? 4) If antecedent, by what mechanism do these factors precipitate or influence the physical disease?

Although the majority of publications about childhood asthma tend to support the psychosomatic thesis, we have chosen to lay most stress on the presumed consequences of the disorder because the chicken and egg, cause vs. effect argument cannot be conclusively resolved without a large, well-controlled, longitudinal study in which all personality characteristics, etc. are carefully documented before the onset of illness. In any case, one of us (P.P.) has argued repeatedly that the relationships are complex and interactive. 'To appreciate the true significance of the psycho-physiologic correlations in childhood asthma, it is necessary to think in terms, not of a unitary psychological factor, but rather of a complex of factors, multifaceted in structure, summative in effect, and mutually interacting.' (Pinkerton, 1971c).

Moreover, as Graham and his colleagues are at pains to point out (1967), 'Clinical impressions, rather than the results of systematic studies, are responsible for the fact that some paediatricians and psychiatrists have come to view the personality of the asthmatic child in terms of a stereotype engendered by a particular type of mother-child relationship.' One explanation for the persistence of such stereotypes (in which the asthmatic child is variously portrayed as anxious, tense, inhibited, shy, intelligent, perfectionist, ambitious, or overly-dependent on an overly protective mother) is that most studies are based on hospital or clinic populations. These we must assume have been selected (in part at least) on the basis of severity, or degree of difficulty experienced by parents or physician in managing the problem.

In an attempt to examine some of these issues using sound epidemiologic evidence, Graham et al. analysed data from the Isle of Wight survey in which sixty-six children with symptoms of asthma in the preceding year had been identified. (An additional ten children had 'probable' asthma.) Features of the child's background (social class), intelligence and educational attainment, together with frequency of psychiatric disorder identified, were compared with children from the sample who had other physical disorders (n = 38), with a group known to be maladjusted (n = 126), and a group of healthy controls (n = 147).

The findings indicate that, in keeping with some of the stereotyped views, the asthmatics were of higher social class compared with other groups. The possibility of reporting bias or the effect of increased mobility might explain this result. The asthmatics also showed a slight but consistent tendency to achieve better results on tests of intelligence and achievement, but there was no evidence of over-achievement. 10.5% of the children with asthma were found to have a psychiatric illness (compared with 6.3% of the controls), the difference being statistically insignificant. However, it was found that the mean number of behavioural symptoms reported by parents and teachers was similar to that reported for children with other physical handicaps; in both cases this was significantly greater than for control children. Some relationship was found with severity of asthma, when disturbed children were compared with those free of psychiatric disorder. Although others have reported that these children are often tense, inhibited and have difficulty in showing emotion, this characteristic — lacking in show of affection — was found significantly more often among the asthmatics only when compared with children with neuro-epileptic disorder but not so when compared with those having other physical disorders.

In summary, the evidence offers little support for specificity of maladjustment among asthmatics, or for its aetiologic import. These findings are in accord with those reported by Zealley et al. (1970) in their study of a random sample of adult asthmatics; with Hahn and Clark, (1967) in their study of the psychophysiological reactivity of asthmatic children; and with those reported by Harris and Shure (1956).

They are also consistent with the conclusions of Neuhaus (1958), in a study in which personality characteristics of asthmatic children were assessed with a battery of tests — The Brown Personality Inventory, The Despert Fables and the Rorschach. Both healthy children and those with heart disease, were used as controls, to test hypotheses about the specificity of disturbance in relation to asthma. The children with heart disease were also compared with a matched normal control group, and both asthmatics and cardiacs were compared to healthy siblings. Such a design has much to commend it, and short of before and after testing, permits the hypothesis to be tested rigorously.

The controls in each case were matched for age, IQ, socio-economic status, religion and number of siblings — a formidable task. The results show clearly that asthmatics were more maladjusted than controls ($p \ll .05$); were more neurotic than controls; and showed more dependency and insecurity, each significant at the five per cent level. However, the children with heart disease were also significantly more neurotic and dependent when compared with controls; yet in neither group were the sick children significantly more disturbed than their healthy siblings! Thus, in spite of the impressive research design, these findings are inconclusive. On the other hand, they do seem to refute any specificity in the nature of disturbance experienced by asthmatic children.

The work of a team of investigators from the Children's Asthma Research Institute and Hospital (CARIH) in Denver, Colorado may shed some light on the continued controversy regarding homogeneity. In the first of a comprehensive series of studies, Purcell and his co-workers (1961) demonstrated some important personality differences between two groups of children with asthma—those who were 'steroid-dependent (S-D)', and whose symptoms tended to persist in hospital, compared with those who improved rapidly following admission to the residential treatment centre ('rapidly-remitting', R-R). A subsequent publication (Purcell and Metz, 1962) related parent attitudes in these two groups to age of onset; and in a third report, Purcell (1963) defined the child's perceptions of the type of stimulus that customarily triggers an asthmatic response. The major finding from this study was that 15 of the 20 R-R children identified some form of emotional arousal with negative affect as a stimulus, whereas only six of the 18 S-D children did so. The findings are interpreted as supporting the hypothesis that 'asthma is more often employed as a learned, defensive-adaptive response by R-R than by S-D children.'

These two sub-groups bear some resemblance to the counter-neurotic, super-stable, non-complaining stoics (S-D), vs. the cossetted, caving-in, neurotically disposed 'invalids' (R-R) referred to by one of us (P.P.) in Section V, p. 192.

In 1965 Clifford compared the two groups to try to identify the connotative meaning of self- and asthma-related concepts by using a modification of the semantic differential technique. He found that there were differences in cognition between the two; the R-R children showed more self-acceptance than those who maintained symptoms. The latter showed less cognitive distance between the concept of asthma and other illness-related concepts, although the results here were less conclusive and appeared to be related to sex.

A more recent and more complex study of the same population is described by Purcell *et al.* (1969) in which the issue of separation from family is distinguished from the effects of removal to a completely different environment and in which the groups are further sub-divided according to their scores on an index of somatic predisposition to allergy (The Allergic Potential Scale). In this investigation the Parent Attitude Research Instrument (PARI) was used with about two-thirds of the parents (mothers and fathers) of the 347 children studied; the asthmatics themselves were assessed through the Children's Personality Questionnaire or the high school equivalent of this test. The results demonstrate clearly the validity of subdividing the population of asthmatic children. Thus, 'A classification comparing high and low allergic potential subjects within the R-R group, showed the largest number of significant differences on both personality and parental attitudinal measures. Greater evidence of psychopathology in children, and undesirable child-rearing attitudes in the parents, was found in the low APS remitters, as compared to the high APS remitters' even though the severity of the disease was identical.

Taken together, these investigations offer abundant support for our assertion that 'asthmatic children do not constitute a homogeneous group.' (Pinkerton, 1970b). Variations in severity of physiological involvement, in parental attitude, and in the child's attitude to his disability, appear to influence not only the therapeutic outcome but the psychological adjustment as well. As the models recently described would seem to suggest, therapeutic success, in terms of stabilization, or prevention of attacks, rather than 'cure', may depend upon providing 'a setting of long-term support by physician, allergist and psychiatrist working in concert to promote realistic acceptance.' (Pinkerton, 1971b).

Throughout the literature on childhood asthma the role of the family in one way or another, is dominant. Nowhere is this more clearly seen than in the study by Dubo *et al.* (1961). Psychiatric interviews with seventy-one children and their families showed no significant relationship between family situation and severity of asthma, but strong relationships between family factors and the child's adjustment at home and at school. The overriding importance of the family in influencing adjustment, but not the basic disease, lends support to our view that emotional factors are a consquence of the disorder, rather than a basic cause.

5. Arthritis

Rheumatoid arthritis has been the subject of many investigations seeking to establish the importance of psychological factors in its aetiology (e.g. Ward, 1971; Moos and Solomon, 1964; Robinson et al. 1971; Moldofsky and Rothman, 1970). The majority of such studies relate to adults, the major exception being the work of Blom and Nicholls (1954) relating to juvenile arthritis. These authors provided evidence that mothers of children with arthritis were pessimistic, displayed excessive guilt and had a masochistic orientation to their role as parents of a disabled child. Although each of these characteristics was more frequent among the parents in question than among those of healthy control children, the authors were unable to prove that they had major aetiological significance, or indeed, that they had even preceded the onset of the illness, since the information was collected retrospectively.

In their final report on this series of studies, they show that the mothers of children with JRA displayed marked depressive reactions to hospitalization; and, more important, that the child was 'depressed, withdrawn, displayed constriction of feelings, was passive and compliant, needed concrete giving to establish a relationship, and was preoccupied with abandonment fantasies.'

Cleveland et al. (1965) and Grokoest et al. (1962) each describe psychological characteristics which they believe are seen frequently among children with rheumatoid arthritis. Cleveland denies, however, that there is any uniformity in the general personality of these children, while Grokoest suggests that they often display 'a chronic, well-masked anxiety state.'

In one of the few controlled studies, McAnarney et al. (1974) showed a consistent pattern of indices of maladjustment that were more frequently found among children with arthritis than among healthy controls. A clinic population of 42 children were examined using a battery of measures. Information was obtained from parents and teachers and tests were administered in identical fashion to the 42 arthritics and their matched controls. Forty-one per cent of the patients had low scores on an index of adjustment reflecting the results of the entire array of measures, compared with similarly low scores in only 29% of the controls.

This finding, while consistent with the hypothesis that more of the arthritics would be poorly adjusted, is statistically inconclusive. Of greater interest and potentially greater importance, is the result of the further analysis which examined the relationship between severity of disability and each of the indices of psychological maladjustment. In only one instance was there a positive relationship, *i.e.* a direct gradation between the three levels of severity (severe-moderate, mild and non-disabled) in the direction predicted. In five other indices, the relationship was linear but negative, that is, the less the disability the greater the maladjustment, and in a further seven indices, a similarly negative but curvilinear relationship was found.

The significance of the results indicates once again that severity of maladjustment is not a direct function of severity of illness but may be inversely related or may be curvilinear: this suggests that two separate mechanisms may operate in relation to severity of illness. On the one hand, those with severe disabilities are more likely to be maladjusted, by virtue of the major restrictions the disorder imposes on their daily lives and the effect it has on the way others behave toward them. On the other hand, the child with mild disorder is in a marginal situation — he is 'unlikely to be regarded as "sick" even though he is constantly reminded through the treatment prescribed and the frequent visits to hospital that he is not in perfect health. Nonetheless he is expected to behave and perform in the same way as his peers.' (See page 171, Section V).

Although no documentation governing the frequency of emotional problems is presented, several papers by Morse (1965, 1966, 1968, 1972) describe the manner in which a comprehensive approach to the arthritic child's care has been organized, and its apparent effectiveness. One paper describes the way hospitalization for the illness was used as an opportunity to stimulate emotional growth, while another describes the parallel roles played in the team approach to the child's care (see page 197, Section V). The potential hazards of teamwork are recognized however and the key to minimizing them is clearly shown to be open communication, both formal and informal. In yet another report, Morse emphasizes the value of involving fathers in the treatment of these children. (To our knowledge this is one of the very few instances in which the role of fathers is recognized, let alone identified, as a salient factor in the care of children with any chronic illness.) One of the goals is to clarify the father's role, since in the care of most children, the major burden and responsibilities rest upon the mother. This potentially inappropriate position is unwittingly enhanced by societal factors making it difficult or unduly costly for the father to attend at most clinic visits. By failing to correct these imbalances, the basic problems of the child are frequently exaggerated, through the additional stress indirectly resulting from fathers being 'outranked,' or 'devalued,' or simply 'neglected.'

That the comprehensive approach described by Morse is effective in minimizing the psychosocial consequences of JRA, is seen in her more recent report (1972), describing the achievements of the 100 patients who had been followed into adolescence or young adulthood. The evidence presented clearly suggests that the majority are doing well scholastically, or vocationally, or at least have high and reasonable expectations. One key to the apparent success is the basically positive and optimistic attitudes shared by the team, combined with the view of the hospital social worker as a 'bridge to community services.' (see page 201, Section V). The picture is not entirely encouraging, however, since Morse comments that unfortunately, 'a case by case analysis indicates some lack of professional understanding that has hampered counselling, discourages students and clients, limited psychological growth, and, in a few cases, even led to detrimental stress.'

6. *Heart disease*

Perhaps more than any other single chronic disease, disorders of the heart have the potential for creating psychological reactions entirely out of proportion to the severity of the lesion. The reasons for this are readily understood. The heart is undoubtedly the organ most commonly linked in the mind of the average person with the maintenance of life. It is steeped in folklore and popular imagery and is, accordingly, invested with tremendous psychological significance. Understandably, therefore, parents are inclined to exaggerate the danger of any symptoms related to the heart and to respond to these misgivings. Predictably, in the circumstances, there has been little difficulty in documenting the consequences of such anxieties and the maladjustment they so often produce.

The simple study by Green and Levitt (1962), for example, was prompted by the disparity so often seen between the physician's judgement of the child's functional abilities and his actual performance. These investigators were trying to determine some of the factors responsible for this 'functional deficit.' They hypothesized that the self-concept of a child with congenital heart disease is constricted when compared with that of normal children. To test their hypothesis, 25 children, eight to 16 years old, were matched with 25 healthy children; each was asked to draw a picture of himself and one of a peer. The height and area of each drawing was then measured and compared for the two groups. The results showed that the self-drawings of the children with heart disease were significantly shorter and smaller than those of the normal children.

This study is no more than a preliminary finding in relation to the basic hypothesis. It is inferred that those with heart disorders have a constricted view of their bodies, and that this was also found in children with intellectual deficits and emotional disorders. It cannot be concluded that the constricted body-image necessarily represents maladjustment, though, as the authors suggest, it may serve as a predictor of future emotional difficulties.

The finding of heightened anxiety among children with heart disease has been reported by a number of investigators. Thomas *et al.* (1970), using questionnaires with both children and their parents, compared the extent of anxiety and other psychological factors shown, with the route of penicillin prophylaxis prescribed (oral vs. intramuscular). They found that 'parents whose children were receiving intramuscular prophylaxis were more protective and more cautious in their estimate of the child's future and that these children showed more evidence of anxiety, whereas those receiving oral penicillin tended to deny or ignore their disease.' About one-third of the 52 children and their parents had been inadequately informed about the disease, or the rationale for the treatment prescribed.

Pursuing quite a different parameter, Barnes *et al.* (1972) set out to assess the degree of anxiety generated by children undergoing open heart surgery. The clinical criteria they adopted were based upon observations and psychiatric interviews. In particular, criteria were used relating to fear of dying, verbalization, motor activity, behaviour, and preparation for surgery, to classify children into two groups: those with severe anxiety and those with mild anxiety. Urinary 17-hydroxycorticosterone levels were obtained at repeated intervals before and after surgery but these were related more to age than to anxiety levels. The findings are interpreted in terms of predicting ability to cope with the stress of surgery.

A similar study by Aisenberg *et al.* (1973) used behavioural observations, interviews, and psychological tests to show that 35 of the 50 children studied responded to catheterization with negative behaviour, or intrapsychic changes, or both; and that the incidence of these reactions increased in the younger child. The importance of these findings lies in emphasizing the need for more adequate preparation for this procedure, or even delaying it, when possible, until a later age.

The studies of Linde and his colleagues (1966, 1970) are among the most definitive in determining extent of maladjustment among congenital heart cases. Although the population studied is unlikely to represent all children with this disorder, in several other respects the approach meets many of the criteria needed for a conclusive investigation. The study group consisted of 98 children with cyanotic congenital heart disease. These were compared with 100 children with acyanotic heart disease of equal severity, 81 normal siblings closest in age, and 40 other normal children. The variables adopted to describe adjustment and maternal attitudes are both well-defined. All the variables were measured using 7-point rating scales, and the results analysed by using t-tests to compare the significance of differences between means and correlational techniques.

The findings, although in some respects surprising, are clear-cut. The most important is that degree of psychological adjustment was unrelated to extent of physical incapacity. In this study, the differences in adjustment between the children with heart disease and the normal controls were significant. The only clear relationships found to be associated with adjustment were aspects of maternal attitude — 'The poorer adjustment of the cardiac child related more highly to maternal anxiety and pampering than to his degree of incapacity . . .' but it is noteworthy that these behaviours 'were significantly greater in the cardiac children than in the normal group and were highest in the cyanotic group.' Not surprisingly, maternal anxiety was related to protectiveness and to anxiety in the child, with little difference in respect of presence or absence of cyanosis. If anything, maternal overprotectiveness (judged by the protectiveness of the physician) is more often found in the acyanotic group.

This phenomenon even applies to children with 'innocent,' *i.e.* non-organic heart murmurs as shown by the study of Bergman and Stamm (1967). In a survey of more than 20,000 school children in Seattle, 75 were found to have no organic heart disease although parents had indicated to the school nurse that the child had something wrong with his heart. Of these, 40% had been restricted in their daily activities and, in the authors' view, most of these unnecessary restrictions were due to the advice given by physicians.

Returning to the studies by Linde *et al.*, they describe in their final report the changes which occur in the functioning of these children over the five-year period of their investigation. It is illuminating that although the differences are small, the mean scores for general adjustment, willingness, self-confidence, and attention consistently indicate that those with heart disease, both cyanotic and acyanotic, are less well-adjusted than the healthy controls. The authors' main interest, however, lies in the differences over time, *i.e.* the changes between first and last tests, particularly for those with and without surgery. Striking improvements were found in most of the adjustment variables in the cyanotic group after surgery, whereas the non-operated cyanotic group showed a significant decline in general adjustment. These changes are paralleled by similar alterations in maternal attitude; and, as with other findings of this nature, it is intriguing to speculate on the causal relationship between these events. The findings are similar to the only other comparable study, an earlier one by Landtman *et al.* (1960), in which the behaviour of 56 out of 84 children was improved following operation.

An annotation in the *Lancet* (1966) aptly summarizes the significance of these findings for the clinician: 'Many lessons can . . . be learned, and the most important of these is an often unsuspected failure of communication. Parents who seem to understand, and say that they understand, all too often arrive home from an outpatient appointment emotionally exhausted and remember little of what has been explained to them . . . The seeds of a cardiac neurosis, once sown, may germinate at a very early age; and in many cases these seeds are planted by the doctor.'

7. *Kidney disease*

Disorders of the genito-urinary tract are common in childhood, by far the most frequent being chronic infections of the bladder (cystitis) or kidney (pyelonephritis). Less common, but of much greater gravity, are disorders such as nephrosis or chronic glomerulonephritis which affect functional capacity and which may, in time, render the organ useless.

In recent years, with the advent of renal dialysis on a wide scale and renal transplantation to a more limited extent, interest in the psychological consequences of these conditions has grown rapidly; the more so in that treatment often involves major ethical considerations, making it essential that emotional repercussions of therapy are understood as fully as possible. What is surprising, however, is the relative neglect of the more common disorders of the genito-urinary system in view of the fact that most psychological theories place heavy emphasis on sexual fantasies. Catheterization of the bladder is a frequent, almost routine step in evaluating these disorders and must be assumed to produce fears of major significance for many children. Yet curiously little attention has been paid to this issue, and indeed, few paediatricians or family doctors involve themselves in the care of children with these disorders once they have been referred to the urologist.

Of necessity, therefore, this section deals exclusively with the psychological sequelae of chronic renal disease. One of the first papers calling attention to this sphere was by Korsch and Barnett (1954), followed by discussion of the specific effects of nephrosis by Korsch and Barnett (1961). This later report was based on the assumption that nephrosis (or any other serious childhood illness) acts primarily as nonspecific stress for both the child and his family. In a prescient statement accurately reflecting our current conceptual model, the authors wrote, 'The age and stage of development of the child, the latent sources of tension in the family, the personalities of the child patient and his parents will determine the psychological reactions to (his) illness to a larger measure than does the nature of the illness itself. In addition, there are certain specific features of any disease which have psychological implications for the developing child and his family.'

The special features of nephrosis which influence psychological responses are its potentially fatal outcome, with or without treatment, and the profound side-effects of therapy with massive doses of corticosteroids. The paper by Korsch and Barnett is a sensitive and detailed discussion of the interactive impact of disease on the family and the child and the potential role of the physician both for good and harm. Drawn as it is from extensive clinical experience, but unsupported by objective data, it adds little however to the basic question of how often such children become disturbed and in what way. On the other hand, it admirably explains the nature of the mechanisms that bring maladjustment about when it does occur. As with other disorders, attention is drawn to the circular relationship between the child's behaviour when he is feeling miserable and the response this evokes from his parents; the role of guilt feelings in both child and parents, and the fear of retribution; the adverse consequences of physical restrictions; the effects of prolonged dependence; the narrowing of social contacts; the effects of painful separations; and above all, the effects of the illness on the developing 'body-image.'

From this essentially clinical description we move to two more recent and systematic examinations of the psychosocial consequences of kidney dialysis and transplantation. The first, by Khan et al. (1971), describes the social adjustment and emotional status, level of intelligence and self-concept of 14 children. Both this and the study by Korsch *et al.* (1973) were prompted to some extent by a thoughtful and provocative paper claiming that the amount of social and economic pressure, physical discomfort and other stresses were hardly balanced by the prolongation of life achieved by these procedures (Riley, 1964).

The data in Khan's study was obtained through both structured and unstructured interviews with the children and their parents, supplemented by the Draw-a-Person test and the results of the WISC. All but two of the children, ranging in age from six to 17 years, were found to be depressed and in several the depression was compounded by denial, anxiety or irritability. Likewise, only one was judged to be well-adjusted socially, while four others were rated 'fair.' The social adjustment of the remainder was either poor or classed as 'getting worse.' Taken together, the results clearly indicate that the majority were having serious social and emotional problems, although it is important to note the authors' admonition that 'some of these problems could have easily been avoided if attention had been paid to the social and family environment.'

Also of interest is that they found the school situation to be 'a major area of concern'; and that some of the feelings of isolation, etc. could have been prevented if the children had been able to attend regular classrooms on days when they were not receiving treatment. Discussion with parents about their expectations for the child is also suggested as a means of counteracting over-protection and excessive sympathy, both of which are common and understandable in these cases.

The other study, described by Korsch and her colleagues, (1973) is exemplary in many respects. The representative nature of the sample and its size are two major limitations, but these shortcomings aside, the project was based upon a variety of subjective, projective and objective measures, and incorporated three control groups. These included matched children with other chronic illnesses from the Rochester random sample previously described; healthy children also taken from the Rochester sample; and 20 children with cystic fibrosis matched for age. The subjects themselves were 35 patients one to five years post-transplantation. In addition to psychological testing, the parents were interviewed using a modification of the Rochester parent questionnaire, plus a new semi-structured interview designed specifically for this study.

Apart from indicating clearly the extent of impact on the family as a whole, the results suggest a high frequency of social maladjustment, increased anxiety, lowered self-esteem, and unusual self-representations in drawings by the children with transplants. Of great interest is the fact that objective tests accurately reflect the presence of psychosocial problems among children already so identified quite independently. These were the children who required psychotherapy and whose clinical situation was frequently characterized by non-compliance.

On the whole, the findings are interpreted as indicating 'good potential for recovery and rehabilitation of child and family after haemodialysis and transplantation.' However, as the authors are quick to point out, in most cases, considerable time has elapsed since the acute phases of treatment, and further, 'continued attention and support was provided for the patients by the comprehensive health care team.' Neither of these factors can be ignored in any future effort to replicate these impressive results.

The need for careful appraisal of the family, the impact of the illness and its treatment on them, and for their active involvement in the treatment programme are similarly stressed by Morse (1974). In addition, Greifer and Barnett (1974) refer to the potentially crucial role to be played by the primary physician in the care of the child with renal disease, if he chooses to remain personally involved. No longer can there be any doubt that successful outcomes such as those described rarely occur if the family is left to its own resources. Much more help is needed and in particular much more needs to be learned about what kinds of help, when it is needed, for whom, and by whom, before psychosocial adjustment can be routinely taken for granted in the care of these children.

COMMON THREADS ANTECEDENT TO MALADJUSTMENT

The findings so far reviewed are of considerable diversity, leading at times to apparently opposite conclusions about the same groups of children. Are the majority of children with haemophilia disturbed, as Agle suggests, or only relatively few, as Mattsson and others have concluded? The same questions may be posed for each of the categories of disorder represented.

Evidence from an ideal study, with before and after measures and case-control comparisons, on samples randomly drawn from the population with a particular illness, is virtually incontestable. But such projects are the exception — in fact, none have been found that meet every one of these criteria. Nevertheless, useful information can be gleaned from less rigorously conducted studies, and even from percipient clinical observations. And when this data is subsumed and found to be concordant, conclusions can be drawn, albeit with reservations. It is therefore, the sum total of the evidence that we examine, and from it, attempt to fashion guide-lines regarding methods of promoting more healthy adjustment to chronic illness.

Although many of the results reported undoubtedly conflict with each other at least in specific detail, some of the more general findings are remarkably consistent. Consequently, each of the following statements is valid:

(1) Among children with chronic physical disorder, most of those studied have a greater degree of frequency of maladjustment than do their healthy peers of comparable background.

(2) Certain features of the disease — its age of onset, manner of progression, prognosis, the type of disability it imposes, its severity and duration — each has a bearing on the likelihood that a child will adjust well or badly.

(3) Some characteristics of the child prior to the illness, especially his intelligence, personality, coping style and any other special assets he may possess — attractiveness, charm, special skills, etc. — are also of importance in predicting his ability to cope with any future chronic illness.

(4) These factors in turn are heavily influenced by the

character of the child's family, and in particular, by the strength, warmth and resilience of relationships that exist within the unit, versus the extent to which the family is burdened by external pressures and stresses.

(5) Within the family, the attitudes of the parents, and perhaps the mother in particular, are of crucial importance. Feelings the parents have about the illness, the effect it has on their lives, and those of the other children, the direct day-to-day burdens it imposes — each of these elements has a direct bearing on the child's coping capacity.

The relationship between the impact of disease on the family, and the impact of the family on the child's self-concept, is circular or 'cybernetic,' in that one affects the other. Clearly, one strategy for intervention is to break into this vicious cycle at one point or another; either by reducing that family's burden, depending on the means available, or by trying to assist the child directly, through amelioration of his handicap, or sublimation of his disruptive behaviour. Ideally, the aim is to prevent the cycle from starting up at all. More often, however, recognition is delayed until problems have already emerged and attempts then have to be made to redress the balance.

The impact of chronic illness on the family has been examined frequently in relation to a wide range of disorders. Table 6 summarizes the principal areas in which adverse consequences have been documented for representative conditions. Unfortunately, measures of family impact are still rudimentary; few studies therefore attempt to do more than catalogue the areas in which problems are reported, and most do so retrospectively — with all the limitations this involves.

Some recent work sets out to examine the dynamics of the situation created by these problems, in an effort to assess how well (or poorly) families cope with their burdens (*e.g.* Klein, 1974, unpublished data). Earlier work by Davis (1963), Farber (1959) and Tizard and Grad (1961) laid the foundations for this approach, but we still do not know enough about the mechanisms whereby families handle the stress of a handicapped child. Hence we are relatively limited in our efforts to help them psychologically. We tend instead to concentrate on minimizing the burdens through more concrete means, such as trying to secure home help for the mother, opportunities for the child to be cared for by others, or arrangements to allow for periods of respite.

Table 6. Problems of families of children with chronic physical illness

Disorders (Author) [N]	Emotional	Marital	Siblings	Social	Genetic	Routines	Financial	Methods
Coeliac (Gardiner, 1972) [28]	*			*				Interview
Tay Sachs (Kanof, 1962) [25]	*	*		*	*			Interview
Asthma (McLean, (1968) [50]			*	*		*	*	Interview
Nephrosis (Korsch, 1954) [20]	*	*						Clinical
Kidney transplant (Korsch, 1971) [87]	*	*	*	*		*	*	Tests
Heart, rheumatic (Glaser, 1961) [25]	*							Interview & tests
Heart, congenital (Glaser, 1949) [25]	*					*	*	Interview
PKU (Keleske, 1967) [16]	*	*					*	Test & questions
Cerebral palsy (Hewett, 1970) [180]	*	*	*	*		*	*	Interview
Diabetes (Crain, 1966) [38]				*				Test & questions
Haemophilia (Mattsson, 1972) [22]	*	*						Test & observation
Cystic fibrosis (Meyerowitz, 1967) [157]	*					*		Interview
Cystic fibrosis (Turk, 1964) [25]		*	*			*		Questionnaire
Cystic fibrosis (Tropauer, 1970) [20]				*			*	Psychiatric
Cystic fibrosis (McCrae, 1973) [100]	*				*			Interview
Spina bifida (Walker, 1971 [107]	*	*	*	*	*	*	*	Interview
Spina bifida (Freeston, 1971) [85]		*				*	*	Interview
Spina bifida (Dorner, 1973) [37]	*	*		*		*		Interview
Spina bifida (Tew, 1973) [59]	*	*						Test & questions
Spina bifida (Richards, 1969) [86]	*	*			*	*	*	Interview
Spina bifida (Hunt, 1973) [77]	*	*				*		Interview
Handicapped (Carnegie, 1964) [600]			*	*		*	*	Interview
Handicapped (Barsch, 1968) [117]	*		*	*	*			Interview & tests
Multi-handicapped (Berggreen, 1971) [20]	*		*	*				Interview
Chronically ill (Cummings, 1966) [60]	*			*				Tests
Chronically ill (Sultz, 1972) [390]		*	*			*	*	Interview

* Problem area documented in study.

The converse aspect of the problem — the attitudes and behaviour of parents toward their disabled child — continues to attract more attention. Psychologists and sociologists alike have tried to determine the extent and manner in which child-rearing is altered when a child has a major physical disability. A superficial review of some of the studies of parental attitudes is provided by Love (1970), whereas Barsch (1968), and Hewett *et al.* (1970) present detailed, systematic accounts of actual child-rearing practices.

Barsch reports on comprehensive interviews with the parents of 177 children who were either blind or deaf, had cerebral palsy or were mongoloid, or suffered from some other 'organic' central nervous system disorder. Hewett's study deals with 180 children under six years with cerebral palsy living in the East Midlands. Parents were also interviewed in great detail about the practical problems of day-to-day living, the effects on family life, problems in education, training and day care, and the extent to which upbringing of these children has been modified because of their illness. (Where possible the questions used by the Newsons, in their Nottingham study, were employed.)

Neither report minimizes the burdens, physical and psychological, experienced by these families. But both, rather surprisingly, emphasize the relatively few ways in which child-rearing itself has been altered. 'The . . . families meet the day-to-day problems that handicap creates with patterns of behaviour that in many respects deviate little from the norms derived from studying the families of normal children. They have more similarities with ordinary families than differences from them' (Hewett). 'These parents gave very little evidence to suggest that any significant changes occurred in their general concepts regarding child-rearing simply because they had a handicapped child . . . They all seemed to have set about the business of rearing the handicapped child according to whatever set of beliefs they held about child-rearing in general . . .' (Barsch).

One cannot examine the phenomenon of adjustment to any chronic disorder without returning repeatedly to a consideration of the central role played by the parents, and the mother in particular. This issue is the theme of a remarkable book by Roskies (1972) in which she describes the 'mothering of Thalidomide children'. Because the author has little to say about the frequency of maladjustment among the small group (20) studied, this commentary may be viewed as a digression, but in our view it is central to the major issue, certainly for the pre-adolescent child.

Roskies relied entirely on a series of structured interviews repeated at intervals over a period of five years. She used the Sears, Macoby and Levin studies as a guide but added many other questions simply because she had a 'hunch' that they might be revealing. In the end, although she views the results in relation to her original aims as disappointing, she appears to come very close to the truth of the matter: '. . . we continuously had the impression of working with a jigsaw puzzle in which many pieces were missing, and where even those that were present could not easily be fitted into an ordered relationship. In a sense, the problem appeared more, rather than less, complex and baffling, as we worked with it.' Some of the difficulty is attributed to the incompleteness and inadequacy of the conceptual model — one that saw the 'problem of thalidomide maternity in terms of the child's partial normality and abnormality, and the mother's reaction to this marginality . . .'

Roskies came to see that the meaning of the child's abnormality was not inherent in the child but rather in the parent's perception of it. And to fully understand this perception required consideration of many other factors — the mother's personality and the social milieu to name but two. Thus, in spite of her disappointment, Roskie is led to the belief that, in the long run, it may be more productive 'to admit the inadequacy of our understanding of the maternity of a handicapped child, than to keep on using approaches whose major distinction is that they provide simple answers to over-simplified questions.'

Certainly the problem is as she sees it: multifaceted, requiring examination from many perspectives. 'If nothing else, this study has confirmed our initial belief that mothers of handicapped children should not be viewed in terms applied to psychoneurotics. The 'acceptance-rejection-overprotection' model has long been proven both theoretically and clinically meaningless, and it is about time that it be given a decent burial. Rather, it is in the psychology of stress, the sociology of deviance, and our understanding of normal developmental psychology that we should seek to understand both the normality and abnormality of this form of mother-child relationship.'

Roskies' comments and conclusions have been quoted at length because they reflect so accurately our own convictions at this point. Having reviewed in some detail the evidence, good and bad, conclusive and merely suggestive, consistent and contradictory, one answer is inevitable: the issue is indeed complex, and no simple model or unitary hypothesis will serve to guide those resolved to promote healthy adjustment among children with chronic disorders. Nevertheless, some guidance is called for, even at the risk of over-simplification, because of our conviction that even the most elementary steps have sometimes been neglected. Accepting that the challenge is both complex and difficult, there is no excuse for clinicians to fail in at least attempting to implement the simple and the obvious.

V

Therapeutic Intervention to Promote Adjustment

Central to chronic handicap of any kind in childhood, whether linked with illness or disablement, is, as we have seen, the basic challenge of adjustment. What this means, what it involves in both the short and longer terms, and how to measure it — each has been allotted detailed review in previous sections. Together, they yield a blueprint for intervention because this is their ultimate import. How best, therefore, to deploy that information to meet the needs of individual children?

DETERMINANTS OF INTERVENTION

Each case is personal; each problem in a sense unique. Yet from the welter of experience amassed by different disciplines, certain elements stand out as basic to the strategy of intervention. Underlying any given programme are five such basic determinants. They are:

(1) the nature of the illness
(2) the child's personal reaction to it
(3) parental and family reaction to it
(4) the therapist's orientation
(5) the attitude of the community

This pentad is equivalent to the triad of contributory factors already attributed to Lipowski (page 28), *i.e. disease-related; intrapersonal;* and *environmental,* which here includes the attitudes of family, community, and the particular therapeutic team.

1. **The nature of the illness**
Over and above the problems common to all disorders in this

THERAPEUTIC INTERVENTION

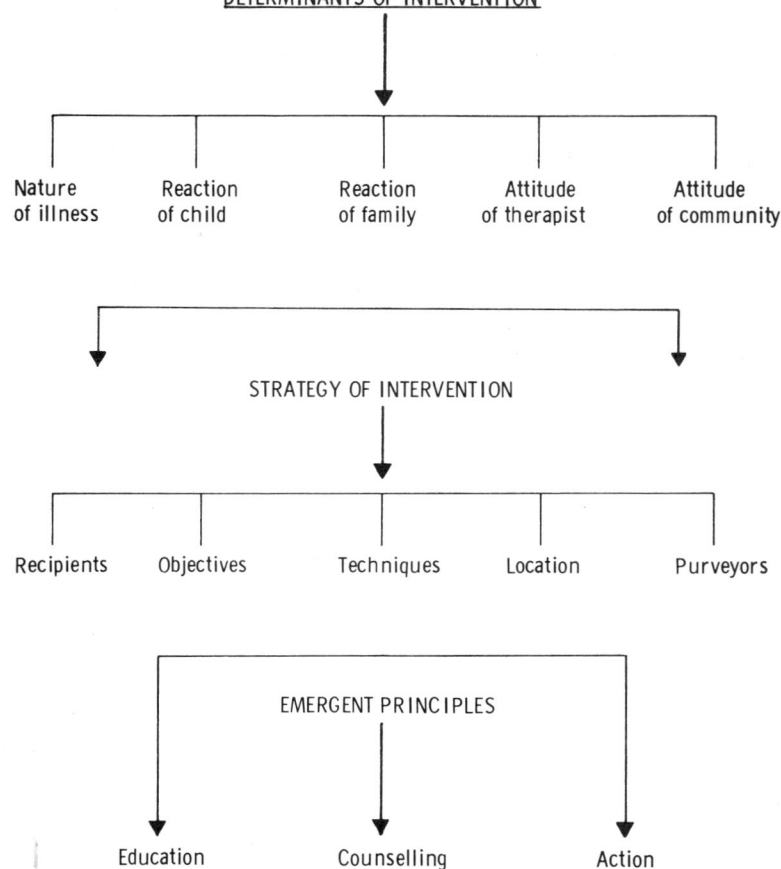

Fig. 4

group — their chronicity, their handicapping potential, and the sense of being different which they engender — the scope and form of intervention may both be influenced by particular properties inherent in the lesion itself. These may be classified as shown in Table 7:

Table 7. Illness characteristics influencing adjustment patterns

Characteristic	Variations influencing responses
Type or site of lesion	locomotor; sensory; cosmetic; communicative
Visibility or stigma	present or absent
Severity of lesion	mild, moderate or severe disablement
Degree of disability	partial or complete
Prognosis	recovery; active; progressive; terminal
Special features	present or absent
Permanence	reversible; life-threatening
Acceptability	aesthetic; rigidity of regime
Age of onset	congenital; acquired early or late
Nature of onset	sudden; insidious; progressive

(a) First the type or *anatomical location.* The study by Rutter *et al.* (1970a), for example, (page 93), demonstrated that, as compared with clinical psychiatric disturbance in the general child population sample, emotional sequelae were three times as common in children with any chronic illness, *e.g.* diabetes, asthma or congenital heart disease; but, significantly, in *neuro-epileptic disorder,* five times as common. Any lesion, therefore, with CNS involvement is particularly likely to give rise to psychological problems. Among these, interference with sensory input, especially defective sight or hearing, or limitation in locomotor function, are obvious examples.

For very different reasons, the acute embarrassment engendered by urogenital anomalies can make for special problems in adjustment. If, in addition, psychosexual orientation becomes an issue, conflict may well reach crisis level.

No less problematic for the teenager with developing heterosexual interests, are the difficulties engendered (say) by ulcerative colitis, especially if it leads to colostomy (Mattsson, 1972). Similarly, cosmetic disfigurement resulting from burns, injury, or unsightly congenital lesion, will pose a particular challenge in overcoming self-consciousness.

The site of the lesion, in other words, can materially affect overall management.

(b) So, too, may its *severity, i.e. the degree of disablement.* On the one hand, serious illness of any kind poses its own particular problems; for example, the congenital heart case with grossly impaired exercise tolerance; the chronic epileptic with frequent and poorly controlled seizures; the child crippled with severe post-meningitic deafness — each has special difficulties with which to contend. However, if the level of disablement should become so overwhelming as to preclude competitive adjustment, and thereby points the need for specialized sheltered provision, paradoxically less conflict may be generated — simply because there is no longer the expectation to cope. Competition has become too unequal, and the indication now is for acceptance of the patient's new role.

It is not necessarily true, therefore, 'that the more severe the . . . disability, the more extensive the psychological problems . . .', a reservation emphasized by McAnarney *et al.* (1974) in their study of 42 children with chronic juvenile arthritis (page 152). Although there was increased incidence of psychological problems among the arthropathied children in general, there was also evidence 'that those with less severe disabilities may be more affected psychologically.'

In other words, it would seem, paradoxically, that the less disabling the lesion and the more marginal its effect, the greater the challenge it may pose for the child in attempting to keep abreast of competitive society. These children are neither so handicapped as to drop out automatically, nor yet well enough equipped to compete on an equal footing. They, therefore, fall between two stools.

This is a point stressed by Cowen *et al.* (1961) in respect to blind children, by Bobrove (1964) in respect of the deaf and by Bruhn *et al.* (1971) for their haemophilic patients. (See also page 153, Section IV).

The marginal case, as thus exemplified, calls in its own way for no less understanding than children more radically crippled. In this sense, marginality and severity represent opposite poles of a disablement spectrum each with its own special problems of management.

Thirdly, certain lesions present problems both for the patient and for his family, by virtue of their (c) *special features*. Consider, for example, highly complex, often life-threatening disorders, with a problematic outcome. Classical illustrations are chronic renal disease involving dialysis or transplantation (Korsch *et al.* 1971, 1973), and major cardiac surgery (Barnes *et al.* 1972). The radical implications associated with such lesions — their drama, threat to life and the major alterations they may induce in body-image — all these are constituent factors affecting overall adjustment. Thereby, they pose a special challenge in their treatment.

Converse implications apply in conditions which are *reversible* in clinical pattern. Childhood asthma is the prime example (Pinkerton, 1974c). In acute bronchospasm, the child is clearly ill — even at times *in extremis*; yet suddenly he can be well again and remain symptom-free for long periods. It is this volatile, unpredictable or capricious element, which makes consistent management so difficult in asthma and generates frustration among parents and doctors alike. No such problem arises with visibly crippling disease — cerebral palsy, cyanotic heart disease, meningomyelocele, etc. Physical treatment of these is stylized because the problem is predictable; whereas in asthma — or migraine, or cyclical vomiting, or epilepsy — the trouble is that between attacks the child can be so well! There are no visible signs of handicap — no calipers, crutches or plaster casts to justify special consideration. In such circumstances, considerable ambivalence can be generated in the most angelic of parents (and in the most tolerant of doctors), with inevitable repercussions for the patient.

Ambivalence affecting the *patient*, on the other hand, is primarily engendered by lesions of rather a different calibre — most appropriately designated, perhaps, as *'unacceptable'*. Such unacceptability derives from two main sources — aesthetic considerations or rigidity of therapeutic regime.

For example, Richardson *et al.* (1961) have demonstrated a gradient of preference among children, both handicapped and non-handicapped, for different types of disability. They found that facial disfigurement and obesity, both visible lesions, rank among the least preferred of physical problems, although neither is intrinsically disabling. Aesthetic bias is thus a factor influencing treatment.

More radical still in implication are the demands imposed by strict adherence to a regular regime in the treatment programme. Diabetes, epilepsy, cystic fibrosis, coeliac disease, haemophilia, all qualify for inclusion in this group, because they share in common the indication for a rigid therapeutic schedule or strict precautionary routine. Adolescents in particular tend to identify such restriction with persisting dependence upon adult authority, which they understandably resent. Hence, one form of rebellion among children with cystic fibrosis, for example, is to sabotage their treatment as a perverse gesture of defiance (Pinkerton, 1969; Tropauer *et al.*, 1970). The same holds true for a proportion of both diabetic and haemophilic teenagers (Mattsson, 1972; Travis, 1974).

This is in fact a highly sensitive area of the chronic illness spectrum, partly because of the tyranny imposed by the treatment regime, but also because it highlights the sense of being different. Personal adjustment thereby becomes the more problematic, and with it the prospects for therapeutic success.

Both the age at which the illness begins (or more particularly the age of the child when it is first diagnosed), and the nature of the onset of the illness, influence the responses of the child and his family in important ways. These have been mentioned previously (see page 162).

More speculative perhaps as a scientific premise are the propositions summarized by Bentovim (1972) to the effect that 'chronic perceptual deficit (in those without brain damage) affects the psychosocial maturation of the child by depriving him of certain experiences essential to his development. For instance, object constancy is a difficult and late achievement in the blind child, and as he remains unsure of the benevolence of those upon whom he depends, he is likely to develop submissive, passive traits.' By contrast, communication difficulties induce a show of temper as the major expression of 'wanting' and impair the child's development of tolerance to frustration. Whether or not such links invariably occur is still open to question, but they do serve to emphasize the role of the disease-specific factor.

2. Personal reaction to illness

Yet, however serious the handicap, however exasperating its capriciousness, or restrictive its treatment schedule, none has any meaning in isolation from the patient himself. 'There is no such thing as sickness', wrote Trousseau, 'only sick people'; in childhood disorder, of course, this concept is further extended to embrace the whole family.

How each child reacts depends, to be sure, upon the kind of difficulties with which he has to contend, thus taking us back to the character of the lesion itself.

Additionally, however, the child's personality, coupled with his level of emotional maturation, are at least two further factors which are bound to influence his overall reaction. This point is made by Lowit (1973) when he stresses that 'Chronic disease . . . varies in its impact with the *developmental stage* at which it first affects the patient.' Similarly, McCollum and Gibson (1970), in their excellent description of family adaptation to the child with cystic fibrosis, describe serial phase-specific responses in the developing child, coupled with crises in management which they potentially evoke. For example, in the toddler, bowel negativism or feeding problems may be encountered as a protest against the unfamiliar positioning necessary for postural drainage; while during infancy, excessive awareness of vulnerability to infection may become a focus of anxiety.

In the four to seven age group, conflict is apparent over prolongation of dependence, sharply crystallized in relation to school enrolment. Two further issues tend to emerge between eight and twelve; they are awareness of, and growing sensitivity to being different, often aggravated by the unavoidably offensive odour of stool; and increased consciousness of the poor prognosis associated with cystic fibrosis.

Finally, during adolescence, there is the emergence of teenage deviance and conflict over the dependence/independence issue, with heightened sense of being different resulting from retarded growth and sexual development.

Predictably, since adolescence is so commonly associated with transient emotional instability, many studies focus attention upon teenage problems encountered in the management of chronic disease. Kohlberg and Rothenberg (1970) for example, analyse in depth the emotional response to multiple life-threatening injuries in an adolescent boy hospitalized for seven-and-a-half months. They demonstrate convincingly the impact of this boy's psychological reaction upon the chequered progress of his rehabilitation.

This theme of teenage rebellion against the iniquities of chronic illness is reiterated repeatedly throughout the literature; for example, by Maddison and Raphael (1971) in respect of diabetes, and by Mattsson (1972) in his admirable review of long-term physical illness in childhood. One such illustration is the resentment felt by epileptic teenagers when they are denied a car driving licence and, therefore, have to tolerate enforced dependence on their parents or friends for transportation.

Similarly, Spencer and Behar (1969) in their study of 26 haemophilic adolescents, cite no less than 46% as showing some form of maladaptation in their search for stable adult masculine identification. This the authors attribute to comparable delay in achieving autonomy, coupled with enforced passivity deriving from the constant danger of bleeding episodes. The problematic behaviour they show may be expressed as learning difficulties in school, lack of educational motivation, antisocial conduct such as vandalism, recklessness and accident proneness, or problems in psychosexual adjustment Again, it is the phase of emotional development which dictates the particular symptom pattern.

Within limits, teenage rebellion is probably a healthier sign than persisting overt dependence. This is a point emphasized by Lowit (1973), but inevitably, in respect of certain diseases, it is bound to make for increased difficulty in maintaining stabilization.

Referring to their own study of 28 haemophilic children and their families, Browne, Mally and Kane (1960) mention the importance of emotional factors in their finding of apparently 'spontaneous' episodes of bleeding, by which they mean non-traumatic precipitants. They imply that conflict situations and the resulting stress derived from them might well act as the equivalent of precipitating factors even though no actual injury is involved. They suggest that the basic conflict in these haemophilic cases is between the child's natural drive to be active and aggressive on the one hand, tempered by his prudent inhibition of that instinct.

More recently, Mattsson and Gross (1966) have investigated in detail the complex problems of the haemophilic child, utilizing a number of parameters. They, too, describe behavioural disturbance as a maladaptive response among the haemophilic boys and youths studied. Within this group, 5 showed a comparable pattern of excessive risk-taking and daredevil activities in apparent defiance of their vulnerable state; the remaining 3 showed a disproportionate degree of dependent passivity.* Again, the same themes of undue compliance versus revolt emerge in these descriptions.

A unique feature of this work has been the application of endocrine studies to psychodiagnostic exploration. For example, using 17-ketosteroid excretion rates as a biochemical monitor, these workers were able to identify two main patterns of psychological adaptation to the challenge of haemophilia (Mattsson *et al.* 1971). Significantly, those patients who seemed to be coping more successfully with the irksome restrictions of the disease, could also be identified by their raised 17-ketosteroid excretion output. In other words, a psychological price has to be paid for better adaptation.

Individual responses to the ink-blot test of body-image boundaries, employed with these same subjects, showed an interesting correlation between relatively successful adjustment, and preservation of a more intact body-image as interpreted by the child himself.

Imaginative work of this kind demonstrates the value of the combined approach — the bio-psycho-social concept (Pinkerton, 1974b) — in attempting to unravel the complexities involved.

It is important, however, to retain a sense of perspective in this, as in every aspect of clinical evaluation. There is encouragement, therefore, in the report by the Mattsson group, that in their series as a whole, improved adaptation does tend to take place with advancing adolescent maturation.

Self-attitude, in fact, is not a static parameter, as we are reminded by Klaus Minde and his co-workers (1972) in their comprehensive study of 41 physically handicapped children and their families. Emotional growth and stronger psychologic defences do go hand in hand with increasing maturation, but concurrently, in the sphere of physical handicap, there comes a growing realization of the sense of difference, and the permanence of that state. Issues are also raised of intrapsychic conflict generated by the child's awareness that he does retain so many 'normal' features, e.g. the capacity to smile like any other child, contrasted with such obviously deviant features as an abnormal gait. There is a price for 'growing up' in any context.

Nevertheless, carefully controlled studies like those by Vignos, Thompson et al. (1972), with rheumatoid arthritic patients, provide a basis for qualified optimism. These workers make an important distinction between the level of disease activity, i.e. the degree of active arthropathy and the level of functional adjustment by the patient in face of disability, i.e. how optimum the deployment of whatever residual function can still be mustered.

In line with almost every other study of this type, the actual level of activity in terms of organic pathology was found *not* to be affected by psychosocial factors; but nevertheless, a gradient of social adjustment could be demonstrated, from optimal to inadequate, in respect of whatever handicap the patient was called upon to tolerate.

In other words, attitudinal factors do make a difference to the overall outcome in chronic disease because they permit a more effective level of response to the rehabilitative programme provided. In this particular study, it was found that patients with higher levels of IQ tended to cope more effectively than those of lower intelligence as measured by objective tests; presumably because the more intelligent better understood the nature of the disease process to which they were trying to adjust. They would thereby be better motivated to cooperate in treatment, and could thus extract more from any given programme than their less fortunate fellows.

The moral of this exercise is that provided patients are intelligent enough to understand what is being done for them, and to benefit from it, social adjustment can be improved by making rehabilitation more comprehensive. Potentially, therefore, the intensity of the care programme does count.

This study of rheumatoid arthritis was undertaken exclusively with adult patients. Clearly, there would be difficulties in trying to duplicate it with arthritic children. While, therefore, it would be unwise to extrapolate by making similar deductions in respect of juvenile arthritis, it is not unreasonable to claim that, with the family as the nuclear unit of treatment, the same principles will apply. This brings into focus the third main determining factor in the strategy of management — the *family orientation*.

3. Parental and family attitudes to the illness

'Thousands of man-hours are expended in the treatment of seizure disorder . . . in the long run, the initial investment of time devoted to exploring the families' attitudes and feelings regarding seizures, results in a saving of time and better seizure control.' (Voeller and Rothenberg, 1973).

These workers are referring to the psychosocial aspects of the management of seizures in children. By this, they do not mean emotional 'triggering' of seizure or psychological self-induction. They refer in fact to commonly occurring lapses in epileptic seizure control attributable in their view to communication problems between the doctor and the family with resulting misunderstanding of instructions, etc. In other words, their experience is completely in line with the observations of Korsch and her colleagues (1968) in their distinguished review of 'gaps in doctor-patient communication.'

Voeller and Rothenberg believe that, in respect of epilepsy at least, 'systematic inclusion of psychosocial dynamics (has) both therapeutic and prophylactic value.'

Their implication of parental attitude as a central factor in effective seizure management, is borne out by Ireton (1969) who claims that 'how parents and others react to a child's (epileptic) seizure largely determines how the *child* reacts and how he sees himself' (over and above the neurologic dysfunction).

What applies to childhood epilepsy applies equally to other chronic childhood disorders. Twenty years ago, for example, Barbara Korsch and her colleagues (1954) were claiming that 'parents who reported the greatest anxiety in their children, were those who themselves voiced the most anxiety, embarrassment and often guilt feelings about their child's illness.' Hence, 'parents' attitude was the determining factor in the child's ability to accept his condition.'

Similarly, Neuhaus (1969) used a battery of attitude skills to systematically study the relationship between 'parental attitudes (mother and father) and the emotional adjustment of *deaf* children.' His experimental group consisted of 84 cases, with the observation that the child's adjustment to his deafness is enhanced by positive, *i.e.* congruent parental attitudes, and conversely, impaired by negative or non-congruent attitudes as between one parent and the other. In his study, he was able to demonstrate that where there is parental discordance, the maternal is on the whole more pertinent than the paternal attitude. Poor psychosocial adjustment, incidentally, was found to interfere with the deaf child's education. In other words, the relationship between the organic substrate (in this case deafness) and the prevailing parental aura, is both reciprocal and highly complex.

This concept of reciprocity is explored by Crain, Sussman and Weil (1966) in respect of their study of diabetic children. Compared with non-diabetic controls, they were able to show through the use of psychodiagnostic instrumental measures, that the development of diabetes in one of the children, by generating intra-family tensions, throws increased strain upon the marital relationship.

The study, in other words, suggests a two-way relationship where chronic illness affects one member of a family group. There is, on the one hand, the potential impact of diabetes upon an already possibly unstable marriage structure; while on the other, intramarital frictions may conceivably contribute to the precipitation of frank diabetes in a predisposed child.

In similar vein, Maddison and Raphael (1971) refer to the increased strain thrown upon parents and siblings by any chronic illness in one of the family. They, too, cite the model of juvenile diabetes.

Indivisibility of the family unit in respect of any crisis with which it may be threatened, is elegantly demonstrated by Gath (1973, 1974) in her detailed study of the siblings of mongol children, and the resulting effect on their behaviour.

Comparable emphasis upon parental attitudes is stressed by Mattsson and Gross (1966) in their extensive survey of the families of haemophilic children. They refer, in particular, to the importance of guilt feeling among certain haemophilic mothers, especially those who feel themselves responsible for the earlier deaths of similarly afflicted male offspring.

As with self-attitude, parental and family attitude is not a static parameter. Making this important point, in the case of physically handicapped children, Minde and his co-workers (1972) stress the changing pattern of parental reaction to handicap as it affects their particular child. They rightly insist that the concepts of 'acceptance' and 'rejection' are both too rigid and too static — they are in fact both subject to constant flux and change — the outcome of parental conflict between a very natural wish for normality in their child, and the bitter realization of his deviance.

McCollum and Gibson (1970) present a similar viewpoint in their study of parental adaptation to cystic fibrosis. They, however, identify a temporal sequence, linked with the progression of the illness. Accordingly, they trace changes in parental attitude through the pre-diagnostic, confrontational, long-term and terminal stages of the condition, relating to them the specific anxieties and stresses associated with each stage.

These diverse references to family involvement in so many different disease entities testify to its key role in successful management throughout the whole range of chronic childhood disorder. Because of their very complexity, however, there is a need for some basic framework within which to evaluate parental and family attitude, in line, if possible, with comparable categorization of self-attitude or self-image in relation to the illness.

Using chronic childhood asthma as a conceptual model, with more than 200 cases as the experimental population, one of us (Pinkerton and Weaver, 1970) felt able to identify 'degrees of acceptance' as the most pragmatic basis for classifying reaction to illness, both in the child and in his family, Roskies' reservations notwithstanding (page 166, Section IV)'. In this model, *realistic* acceptance is taken as the optimum, differentiating, for each child, what he can *reasonably* hope to achieve from what would be unrealistic in respect of degree of handicap involved. On this foundation, the range of attitude may be held to extend from over-acceptance, on the one hand, *i.e.* over-investment in the illness, to non-acceptance, or denial of handicap on the other.

So far as the patient is concerned, over-acceptance tends to be associated with immature, hypersensitive or neurotic personality profiles; non-acceptance with more robust personality structure, tending toward stoicism, or even a more active attitude of revolt. Within limits, refusal to concede may be wholly commendable; but if it can only be sustained through risking serious further impairment in physiological function, *e.g.* as in asthma, diabetes, or cystic fibrosis, then surely the price is too high! Patently, therefore, the balance is a delicate one, varying from child to child, and hovering between unrealistic denial of obvious danger signals on the one hand versus hypochondriacal self-indulgence on the other — a highly individual formula for the child as well as for his family toward the illness in question.

It is important, moreover, to confine it to the immediate problem, *i.e.* to avoid 'contamination' which might lead to preferential treatment, or constriction of personal responsibilities. Living within whatever limitations the disorder may impose means physiologic rather than psychologic limitation.

An equivalent attitude spectrum is applicable to the parents of these handicapped children. On the one hand, over-acceptance (or over-involvement) leads to cossetting over-protection and thereby, perpetuation of dependence, as exemplified by Linde *et al.* (1966) in relation to congenital heart disease, (page 157) and by Mattsson and Gross (1966) in connection with their haemophilic studies. Non-acceptance, on the other hand, is associated with ambivalence or even frank rejection on the part of parents. Admittedly, these attitudes are experienced with varying intensity; they rarely remain static. In practice, therefore, we can only concern ourselves with the prevailing parental aura as it emerges during clinical evaluation; but if, in this sense, it is sufficiently sustained, it will, in time, either erode the child's self-image and thereby undermine his stability, or conversely induce revolt among children of tougher mental calibre.

To some extent parental attitudes are shaped by the character of the illness itself, *e.g.* heart disease tends by and large to evoke an aura of protective supervision. On the other hand, any suggestion of congenital stigma, physical or mental, associated with the lesion, sometimes generates hostile feelings, especially in the father, because of its implication of a slight to his virility.

Clearly, therefore, attitude formation has a multifactorial basis. Contributing to it are the personalities of the parents themselves, their respective personal backgrounds, and the character of other relationships within the family, whether tension-free or tension-ridden. The essential feature in all this is whether corporate reaction is supportive or critical in character.

These considerations point the way to rational therapy, based first upon an evaluation of family interaction, *i.e.* positive, opting out, or hostile; and secondly, upon the family's level of tolerance to chronicity and progression of the illness under review.

4. The therapist's orientation

Intervention, however, involves the therapist and his attitudes no less than those of the patient and his family. Success, in fact, may hinge as much upon the orientation of those conducting treatment as upon those receiving it. Just as positive concern enhances the prospect so a negative attitude can detract from it, even to the point of sabotaging prognosis. Whatever the lesion, therefore, personal involvement on the part of the therapist, over and above his professional expertise, is an essential ingredient in the strategy of intervention. Yet all too often the doctor may not even be aware of this important aspect.

In other words, much depends upon the therapist's interpretation of what treatment entails, *i.e.* how comprehensive (or circumscribed) his concept of the scope of therapy. Attitudes range from the narrow standpoint of purely technical intervention to the all-embracing concept of global intervention, which involves the family, the unit staff, and the essential links with community services. The organization of the renal dialysis unit represents the classic model for the study of these contrasting attitudes (Kaplan-De-Nour, 1971) as confirmed by Korsch et al. (1971) and by Wolters et al. (1973). Percipience among paediatricians still varies profoundly with respect to non-technical aspects of children's handicaps and the role they themselves play (unconsciously) in furthering or retarding adjustment, through their personal orientation. For too many doctors problems of adjustment still have to reach too manifest a stage before they are recognized as such and properly dealt with. There is, therefore, a need, among doctors and nurses alike for enhanced awareness of impending failure to adjust, together with increased skill in recognizing prodromal signs, so that corrective measures may be instituted earlier with correspondingly better prospects for success.

5. The attitude of the community

Professional attitudes may be tempered in turn by attitudes within the wider community; but by the same token, treatment advances can often educate public opinion toward a more enlightened outlook. This is a two-way process of influence. Whichever way it operates, community factors undoubtedly dictate the range of options available for intervention, depending on prevailing culture and local traditions.

In England, for example, as estimated by Court (1971), one-third of families feel isolated upon transfer to new housing estates despite enhanced material facilities. If this applies to presumably intact family cells how much more applicable is the threat of isolation to handicapped children and their parents, already conscious of feeling different? (Grantham, 1971).

By contrast, Williams (1973) draws attention to the tolerance and humanity shown in less sophisticated cultures toward handicap in their midst — because they still believe that all, however humble, may contribute a little to the common good. Making a plea for similar enlightenment in our modern urbanized society, Helsel (1967) emphasizes the value of encouraging 'the dependent handicapped to be part of our society — a society that so badly needs what they have to teach; compassion, understanding and respect for the dignity and worth of every living creature.'

Yet in practice, as she points out, widespread prejudices still persist among these self-same handicapped against making use of those facilities which are available — such is their misgiving about charitable overtones; so that however comprehensive the provisions their proper operation depends upon overcoming suspicion in the users.

It depends, too, upon another factor — community coordination. But, so often, according to Helsel, the converse applies, *i.e.* manifest incoordination, so that services for the physically handicapped are fragmented and lacking in uniformity, with resulting confusion and less than adequate utilization.

The lesson is clear: enlightenment is not enough. Not only must there be the forward looking element in community attitudes necessary to promote effective intervention, but to insure its optimum impact delivery of care must be organized and integrated with insight.

Nowhere is this more apparent than in the field of special education, provided under school health regulations in England, for various categories of handicap. One of us had made this the subject of special study (Pless, 1969). What emerges is that legitimate referral for residential schooling on strictly medical grounds is undoubtedly of benefit in certain cases, *e.g.* for stabilizing asthmatics or diabetics who might otherwise drift into progressive organic deterioration. All too often, however, 'the central reason for seeking placement was (not medical, but) the presence of a severe behavioural problem.' There was in fact a lack of any discernible consistent referral pattern among local education authorities seeking to accommodate children with chronic handicap. Rather did it seem their policies were governed by expediency, *i.e.* 'in part simply by the availability of special schools . . . (or) by economic reasons, or by the extent to which they failed to use their social workers and counselling resources in a preventive and supportive fashion.'

In short, like Helsel's criticism of incoordinate services for cerebral palsy in the United States, the plea by Pless *et al.* is against 'the indiscriminate use of boarding for the physically handicapped child (in England), and the absence of any systematic critical evaluation of its appropriateness for the task at hand.'

Quite independently, based upon entirely different case material, the same conclusion was arrived at by the co-author in his own study of chronic childhood asthma; because this brought to light similar anomalies in rationale for long-term residential placement (Pinkerton, Weaver and Henry, 1971a).

What applies to handicapped children as potential pupils in special schools equally applies to them socially. While lip service is paid to the importance of integrating them into 'normal' society, the need to protect them from stigma is still adduced as a reason for segregation or special placement (Dibner and Dibner, 1971). Yet these authors have clearly shown, in a series of summer camp field studies, exploring interaction between handicapped and non-handicapped children, that 'type of disability was not related to adjustment.' What mattered most in keeping up at camp was social maturity, degree of independence and capacity to participate in majority activities despite physical limitations. That this could be achieved by certain children irrespective of the nature of their handicap establishes two points; first that integration *can* be successful and does have positive value; and second, where it fails to succeed, the explanation lies not in the lesion itself, but in psychosocial maladjustment which curtails capacity to cope. The implications for community action are obvious.

But why is such practice currently so fragmentary? One explanation is offered by Davis (1974). 'Patterns of health care in (our Western) society . . . are structured so predominantly (on) . . . "the acute illness model" (that) the chronically disabled . . . come inexorably to assume the status of a "residual category" . . . and even where (they) . . . "qualify" for the necessary social and human services . . . these tend to be, if not actually unavailable . . . meagre, fragmentary, remote and unco-ordinated — again testifying to the fact that services for the chronically ill constitute a kind of "afterthought".'

To recapitulate, therefore, therapeutic intervention, if it is to succeed, must take cognizance of all five determinants —

the illness itself and its particular features, the attributes of the child, the characteristics of his family, the resources of the physician, and the milieu of the community.

THE STRATEGY OF INTERVENTION

Assuming optimum account of the above components, how best to forge them into programmes of management appropriate to individual circumstances? To this end, five further interlocking factors are involved. They are:

1. WHO most warrants treatment and in WHAT order of priority?
2. WHAT are the therapeutic objectives, and WHEN should they be optimally timed?
3. HOW are they best carried out, *i.e.* by WHICH techniques?
4. WHERE is the optimum location for treatment?
5. By WHOM should they be provided?

1. The recipients of intervention and their order of priority

By and large, prospects for successful intervention are directly related to how effectively the family can be involved. The more fragmented the approach the less favourable the prognosis. 'It is necessary to think of the handicapped family rather than just the handicapped child. It is essential therefore that the analysis should not be confined to the nominal patient . . .' (Goldie, 1966).

In other words, in management, as in adjustment, the family is indivisible — as a general rule, though not invariably.

There are undoubtedly occasions when family cohesion is unattainable. There may be overt disruption of family ties, with frank rejection of the patient because he creates yet another problem; covert marital tension which militates against solidarity of support; or perhaps sickness in one parent which prevents his or her more active involvement.

In any of these situations, the only pragmatic option available may be to focus on the child himself and try to compensate him for what is lacking in his own domestic circle, that is, to rehabilitate him in spite of his family.

(Alternatively, the plan of treatment may specifically call for focus on the patient with deliberate exclusion of family contact — at least by the same therapist. (Especially is this so for adolescents who commonly resent any sharing of the problems as an affront to their emerging independence.) For example, Spencer and Behar (1969), describing conflicts which beset adolescent haemophiliacs, emphasize the value of brief psychotherapy exclusive to these vulnerable young people through the medium of a medical authority in whom they trust.

Individual versus group selectivity
Over and above this issue of individual *selectivity* in planning treatment, priority considerations equally apply to certain *groups* of patients. By no means all children with chronic illness encounter psychosocial difficulties that warrant intervention — some are known to cope more effectively than others because the level of family functioning is superior; conversely, the poorly functioning child or family constitutes a relatively higher risk in terms of coping potential, with correspondingly greater prospect of adverse emotional repercussions (Pless *et al.*, 1972).

Fig. 5 illustrates schematically the gradation of 'risk' for child and family and its relationship to level of intervention recommended for optimal benefit, or any benefit. Since few, if any, localities enjoy so generous an allotment of resources as to effectively meet the needs of *all* categories of risk, care must be taken to husband available resources in order to deploy them most effectively overall.

The zones A to E shown in the figure represent increasing levels of 'risk' for the child, based on child or family characteristics. Children in zones A or B are those regarded as being at 'low risk' because of their own strengths and assets, those of their families, or both. Conversely, children in zones D and E must be regarded as being at 'high risk' for maladjustment and, as the figure suggests, a very large amount of resources would be required to obtain any benefit. Thus an optimal allocation of resources in order to maximize results across all risk groups would require that some children in zone D and most in zone E receive little intervention in those communities where such services can be distributed rationally and with foresight. Instead these services might most profitably be utilized, as shown, for those large numbers of children whose risk levels are, in effect, 'intermediate'.

This means avoiding the temptation to concentrate exclusively on high-risk families at the relative expense of those less obviously in need of intervention. To the extent that problem families remain a prime priority they must never be neglected; but a point can be reached where the response achieved is so questionable relative to intensity of effort put in, as to raise the issue of alternative redeployment.

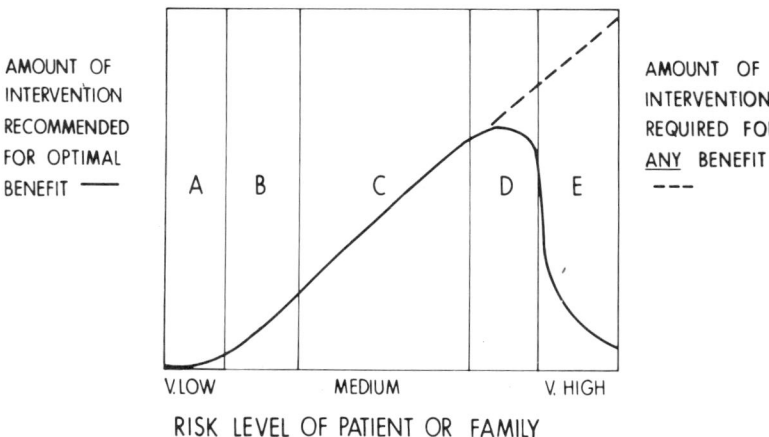

Fig. 5

Focus on more moderate risk levels at an earlier stage in the evolution of adjustment may conceivably have a prophylactic effect, thereby, in the long run, reducing escalation of demand. Calculating this gradation of need against the expertise available is an important aspect of intervention policy.

2. The objectives of intervention and their timing

The overall goal of management must surely be acceptance of irreducible restrictions without over-acceptance — clearly a prescription tailored to the individual child. Yet within this global formula certain shifts in emphasis can be identified between one disorder and another and even between different stages of the same disorder.

For example, 'for parents of retardates, *understanding* as much as possible about their child's mental retardation appeared to be a major goal, whereas among parents of fibrocystic children, major emphasis is laid upon their child receiving *treatment* (Blumenthal, 1969). Both conditions generate profound parental guilt, but while vigorous therapy of cystic fibrosis helps to counteract the family's sense of helplessness and so assuages guilt, there is no comparable prospect for retardation as yet. For these parents, therefore, once that reality is grasped detailed information provides the key to reassurance — that everything possible is being done for their child notwithstanding, and more important, that they are not personally culpable. Similar considerations apply to parents of leukaemic children. They, too, must feel convinced that nothing is being neglected that offers conceivable hope before they can begin to come to terms with so threatening a challenge.

Detailed briefing or explanation in fact is an important component of managing any chronic disorder — the more problematic the outcome, the more vital this indication. 'No substitute has been found for facing up to, and understanding the problem (of handicap or chronic illness) objectively at an early age.' (Bleck and Headley, 1961). This is not to decry however the complementary value of ventilation (page 195).

Endorsing this point, Maddison and Raphael (1971) explain that 'in children, the realistic restrictions imposed by illness, however bad . . ., are almost always less crippling than the fantasy ones constructed by parents and child . . . The more factual the knowledge . . . imparted, the better . . . to both mother and child.'

Hence the prime value stressed by Kennell *et al.* (1969) of educating parents of children with rheumatic fever in the basic medical facts of the disease. Their research highlighted the extent of factual ignorance and the gross level of misconception among parents regarding the disorder. Nor is it only the parents who repay such tutoring. The children too can benefit specifically in that some were shown to harbour unwarranted fears of death through non-existent cardiac involvement.

The temporal factor
Imparting information however is not a static process. For one thing, as McCollum and Gibson (1970) have shown (page 174), in relation to cystic fibrosis, differing facets of management assume overriding significance at various stages of the disease; and for that matter at different ages — calling for corresponding modification in briefing procedure. The same holds true for other comparably disabling disorders.

But even at a given point in the natural progress of the illness, 'timing is important . . .; information may create unmanageable anxiety if . . . imparted (too early), though the more common error is to leave it too late, or to give inadequate or ambiguous messages (or none at all!)' (Maddison and Raphael, 1971).

But whether imparted early (preferably), or late, medical briefing about the disease will almost certainly have to be repeated, again and again, if its unpalatable implications are to be absorbed (Blumenthal, 1969). This same phenomenon of 'delayed registration' is touched on by Wood *et al.* (1967) in their discussion of psychosocial factors in phenylketonuria, 'Time' — they say — 'is needed to work through (the significance of the data)'.

Smithells (1969) summarizes the point succinctly in his reference to counselling in congenital anomalies. 'On the first interview at which the news of the defect is broken, little of what is said is remembered but the telling makes a deep impression.' The same theme is propounded by one of us in discussing parental acceptance of the handicapped child and how best to promote it (Pinkerton, 1970a).

Yet with all this insistence upon facing facts and being frank with the patient and with his family, sight should not be lost of the need for optimism. In a thoughtful study of cerebral palsied children and their parents, Keith and Markie (1969) compared the estimates of handicap as assessed by individual parents with those of the personnel actually involved in management. They found that as a group the parents tended to over-estimate their child's potential relative to professional judgement — a predictable finding perhaps but not necessarily to be deplored. On the contrary, so long as parents are expected to cope, some degree of bias is no bad thing, even at the sacrifice of strict realism. In short, we should try not to rob the parents of their prerogative to hope. After all, they have to live with the problem — we only have to consult about it.

Are we then to infer that the object of intervention is purely to help families to live with their special burden as equably as they can, while they preserve a realistic outlook? Is nothing more involved in the exercise? — far from it. There are practical derivatives of this philosophy which are of potentially major import. They may best be illustrated by further reference to the model of childhood asthma (Pinkerton, 1974a).

Starting from the premise that self-attitude and family attitude materially affect both therapeutic response and prognosis (pages 174-8), a formula can be constructed for estimating their composite degree of influence. It is based on the contention that asthma is not a homogeneous entity pathophysiologically. It has in fact a wide spectrum of severity as measured by tests of ventilatory function. This means that for any given grade of ventilatory impairment clinical problems are to be anticipated in proportion, which allows comparison with the prevailing symptom complex. Thus, minimal levels of impairment should be associated with equally minimal and insignificant symptoms, while severe involvement should produce maximum crippling effect — with gradation of response between. Where, therefore, significant discrepancy is encountered between pathophysiological severity (as monitored objectively) and the degree of obtrusion of presenting symptoms, the possibility of psychologic overlay should always be suspected — in either direction. That is, where the prevailing aura is over-accepting, subjective symptoms tend to be disproportionately troublesome, whereas in non-acceptance, symptoms tend to be disproportionately suppressed — in both cases relative to known degree of ventilatory impairment.

In the first case, there is needless restriction of activity, *i.e.* an exaggerated, caving in, or invalid response; while in the second, there may be dangerous denial of whatever limitations are imposed by the lesion, even to the point of fatal outcome (Pinkerton, 1971a).

Incidentally, most studies in psychosomatic correlation have emphasized the role of neuroticism in producing functional exaggeration of symptoms (*i.e.* over-acceptance). Less attention has been focused on the potentially more hazardous significance of the counter-neurotic or 'super-stable' personality profile associated with non-acceptance (Pinkerton, 1973). The point is that these children and their parents appear so disarmingly 'normal' as to detract from any suspicion of psychodynamic overlay; yet the super-stable or stoical group, by denying legitimate symptoms, may be much more 'at risk' than the traditionally 'neurotic' group.

This is the principle of *symptomatic concordance* (Fig. 6). It applies not only to asthma, but to other disorders in which there is a comparable spectrum of pathophysiological involvement equally accessible to objective measurement, *e.g.* heart disease (monitored by exercise tolerance or cardiography); cerebral palsy (reflected in demonstrable locomotor impairment); diabetes (glucose testing results); or epilepsy (serial EEG tracings).

Given disproportionate presenting symptoms in any of these conditions, pathology of attitude, whether over-accepting or non-accepting, is worth exploring as a possible 'contaminating' factor. Correcting it may make all the difference to stabilization of the organ system involved. In such circumstances, the goal of realistic acceptance becomes more than academic in significance — it assumes very real pragmatic importance.

3. Techniques of intervention

How best then to achieve this objective? A range of techniques has been described, extending from direct intervention with the child himself, by dint of various procedures, to involvement of the parents in different ways, with intermediate steps between these two approaches. No single exercise commands a monopoly. On the other hand, similarities in technique keep cropping up between one set of workers and another, despite their independence of each other — testifying in a sense to the validity of procedures they advocate in common.

PRINCIPLE OF SYMPTOMATIC CONCORDANCE

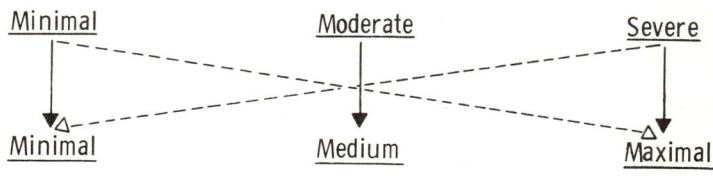

———▶ Symptomatic concordance ie. "adjustment"

------▷ Symptomatic discordance ie. "maladjustment"

Fig. 6

Direct intervention with the child
The use of social group work clubs, for example, is urged by Kolodny and Waldfogel (1967) as a means of trying to integrate physically handicapped children with their non-handicapped peers. Thereby, they argue, intergroup tensions stand to be reduced by removing on the one hand,

misconceptions about handicap (so elegantly demonstrated by Richardson — see page   ); while curtailing on the other, the tendency for their concealment by the affected children themselves.

Grantham (1971) pursues a similar theme in her advocacy of pre-school play group facilities to be extended to handicapped children.

An entirely different modality — important because so readily overlooked — is the role of physical procedures in promoting emotional adaptation. These include surgical, endocrine and physiotherapeutic measures.

Solow *et al* (1974), for example, make reference to improvement in 'mood, self-image, ego-strength and vocational effectiveness' as a consequence of intestinal by-pass surgery for severe obesity in their series of 29 young adult patients. Similarly, Knorr *et al.* (1968) in a 10-year survey, describe the psychosocial implications of cosmetic surgery in adolescence. They rightly emphasize the preoccupation of adolescents with physical appearance and body changes, their sensitivity, but *pari passu*, their enhanced propensity for response to relatively minor modifications — evidence the gratifying results of rhinoplasty, mammaplasty, otoplasty, and dermabrasive procedures for acne, as practised by the group.

In relation to their treatment of Klinefelter's syndrome with testosterone enanthate, Johnson *et al.* (1970) refer to the improvement in body-image, sex drive, and assertive masculine behaviour incidentally achieved, and elegantly monitored by them through the medium of serial Draw-a-Person sketches undertaken by their subjects.

Physiotherapy has a comparable role to play in enhancing self-image among juvenile asthmatics through specially formulated programmes of physical fitness (Petersen and McElhenney, 1965; Hyde and Swartz, 1968).

Yet another therapeutic approach is made possible, in conditions such as asthma, through their clinically reversible patterns (page 172) — namely, the behaviour modification techniques. The classic research in this field has been the work of Creer and his colleagues. They have demonstrated convincingly one method of 'extinguishing' manipulative overlay or invalid tendencies, and even improving peak expiratory flow rates, in childhood asthma, through the practice of behaviour therapy procedures (Creer, 1970; Creer and Yoches, 1971; Alexander, Miklich and Hershkoff, 1972).

For epilepsy, which is similarly mercurial in its clinical pattern, Ireton (1969) describes an alternative version of behaviour modification technique addressed this time to the control of conduct difficulties in pre-school or infant class epileptic children. He advocates coaching their teachers in 'systematically rewarding (positively) adaptive behaviour.'

As in all such definitive programmes, however, there is invariably a bonus 'spread' of positive repercussions affecting other aspects of management — in other words, no single avenue of approach is indisputably the 'right' treatment.

For instance, the opportunity to ventilate fears or resentments generated by chronic illness or handicap is unquestionably of equal value in overall management. 'Adequate medical care must also provide an opportunity for the child to ventilate his own anxiety and anger; opportunities for self-expression through play are invaluable in this regard.' (Maddison and Raphael, 1971). Yet in a sense, this property of 'release' is diametrically opposite to behavioural 'control'. In practice there is room for both types of procedure and for that matter, many more.

Ventilation indeed is of paramount importance for children and their parents alike in this area of intervention; but as Martin (1967) comments, in respect of adult coronary care, 'the mere giving of information about the illness may not (of itself) reduce the tremendous anxiety created (by its life-threatening implications)'. Tutoring (educative) and ventilation (off-loading) really exert a complementary effect as classically demonstrated in the hospital treatment of children with rheumatic fever researched by Rie, Boverman *et al.* (1964). In practice, the techniques tend to be combined, often intuitively, by the clinician. The brief psychotherapy described by Spencer and Behar (1969) for example utilizes elements of both.

But theirs is a didactic model, whereas alternative techniques might prove equally effective, especially with this same age group. The more 'open' group discussion type of therapy, for instance, has much to commend it and was indeed presaged 20 years ago for diabetic teenagers by Korsch et al. (1954). Summer camp experience for juvenile diabetics (McCraw and Travis, 1973) constitutes a more recent innovation along the same lines. Group counselling in fact may also provide a bridge across which to introduce procedures for parental involvement.

Programmes of parental involvement
What applies to direct intervention applies equally to parental involvement — the same components contribute to both and complement each other.

Thus, more than 20 years ago, Milman (1952) was advocating the role of group therapy with parents in promoting rehabilitation among their physically handicapped children. He chose to stress the value of reducing isolation by encouraging these parents to exchange views and to compare experiences in coping with the problem. In the same period, Korsch and her colleagues (1954) were devoting fuller attention to this same theme. Their emphasis was on providing information (about nephrosis, diabetes, etc.) to parents — the educative factor — without curtailing scope for ventilation, including ventilation of negative feelings against certain doctors. They cautiously stipulate however that theirs is not the classical group psychotherapeutic approach. 'Group therapy may arouse parental anxiety about the seriousness of the illness, hitherto not expressed and perhaps difficult to control or defend.' They still adhere therefore to the didactic model, believing that to discard medical authority 'tended to unnerve the parents'.

Nevertheless, there is clearly scope for alternative techniques, and in the intervening years, each has attracted its own protagonists. Linder (1970), for instance, describes the opposite of the didactic model — the development of cohesion within a small group of mothers of handicapped children — where there was no formal leader, no tutoring, and no direction. The evolution of 'strength' was quite spontaneous, through mutual exchanges and support.

Wright (1970) actually classifies four different approaches to parent counselling including his own version of installing the parent as 'the agent of change.' Among other techniques described, many differ more in detail than in basic principle; in practice, much depends on the time and therapeutic skill locally available. Pertinent in this respect (page 94) is the value of utilizing lay persons as family counsellors in protecting chronically ill children from developing secondary psychosocial handicaps (Pless and Satterwhite, 1972). The modest financial outlay involved in this project is in inverse ratio to the encouraging results achieved, as confirmed by the families who actually took part in the counselling programme.

Admittedly, there are polarities of emphasis — tutoring vs. ventilation, medical vs. non-medical, unstructured vs. structured. Irrespective of orientation, however, the basic value of counselling seems indisputable, as witness the endorsement by Cowie (1967) for spina bifida, Taft (1973) for muscular dystrophy, or Mattsson and Agle (1972) for haemophilia.

McCollum and Gibson (1970) describe perhaps the best compromise in their composite programme of work with the parents of fibrocystic children. They advocate a three-tiered plan beginning with medically orientated consultation about management — only practicable therefore with medically qualified personnel, the objective being educative; going on to group discussion at which both paediatrician and medical social worker are available but not dominant and in which there is exchange of views fostering mutual support and countering isolation; going on, in turn, to individual interviews where appropriate, with the medical social worker, to examine in greater depth and in private, the origins of anxieties thrown up by the group without threatening the defences of other parents.

4. The location of intervention

Basically, the choice lies between hospital, special school and community-based facilities. Each has its special indications and advantages but each is also open to misuse. Defending hospital admission as a potential 'growth' experience for rheumatoid arthritic children whose condition warrants in-patient management, Morse (1965) comments that by including parents, *i.e.* supporting them psychotherapeutically, taking the load of nursing off them (and hence reducing their guilt), and demonstrating physical techniques of therapy — in other words, mounting a multi-disciplinary staff approach — the dangers of emotional deprivation can largely be countered — so making a virtue out of necessity. The pioneering nature of Morse's work has already attracted comment (page 153).

The same motivation prompted Green and Durocher (1965) to set up a hospital-based parent education project aimed at 'improving parent care of handicapped children through demonstration, instruction, guidance and support,' organized by a specially engaged professional team member — such in their experience was the extent of locally existing deficiencies.

Most models of this kind, paediatric in their orientation, are largely outpatient services predicated on the need for specialized surveillance or treatment — biochemical, electronic, physiotherapeutic or bio-engineering — required by the patient to monitor his particular systemic dysfunction, and not readily available elsewhere.

However, Mildred Creak (1971) regards the busy teaching hospital ward, with its restricted space and technical devices, as unsuitable for comprehensive management of disorders such as childhood asthma. These respond better, she feels, in a less intense, more 'convalescent' milieu.

One such service has been described by Bernstein and his colleagues (1960) for 'juvenile intractable asthma.' Their rationale is the combination, on the spot, of group therapy for parents with comprehensive paediatric, psychologic and educational facilities for children, available on campus and provided under one roof by a coordinated professional health team. As opposed to Peshkin's nationally-based concept for the treatment of childhood asthma (1930) which made for so much difficulty in sustained follow-up, this local provision facilitates both continuity and contact with the family.

Despite the prevailing trend toward community-based services — a movement which we unequivocally support — there are still circumstances in which admission to hospital remains the recommendation of choice. These indications have been described elsewhere by one of us (Pinkerton, 1974a). They include:

1. Diagnostic clarification of the clinical picture.

2. Planned separation between conflicting family factions.
3. Boosting the morale of patients (and their parents) with unrelievedly chronic handicap, by sharing their burden.
4. The concrete demonstration to doubting parents that improvement can be achieved by means of stable and consistent management.

Nevertheless, for the longer-term rehabilitation of some forms of chronic illness, residential schooling may well be preferable to the long-stay hospital. Much depends upon the severity of the condition, the degree of difficulty in maintaining stabilization as in, for example, diabetes, asthma or epilepsy, the domestic circumstances, and the social milieu. Misuse of the facility has already been mentioned (Pless *et al.* page 184), and therefore care must be exercized in recommending it. As a general rule, if pathophysiological considerations permit, the aim should be to keep the child at home and certainly not to place him residentially for reasons of objectionable behaviour — that *is* a misuse of the boarding special school.

Keeping him at home, however, need not mean denial of therapeutic provision. For example, Bleck and Headley (1961) advocate a pre-school nursery programme for cerebral palsied children, which includes active parental involvement and counselling. For the older child, McCraw and Travis (1973) demonstrate the boosting effect on juvenile diabetics of attending a special summer camp, using self-esteem and manifest anxiety as the measured parameters of change. Much earlier, Holden (1962) had described comparable changes in body-image, as monitored by the 'Draw-a-Person' test (p.54) among physically handicapped children introduced to summer camp experience.

An intriguing innovation has been described by Booth (1965) in which residential weekend courses were arranged for families of cerebral palsied children, with encouraging improvement in outlook and coping, confirmed at follow-up enquiry.

On the other hand, as noted earlier (page 150), Purcell *et al.* (1969) have elegantly demonstrated the converse by procuring predictable improvement within a group of asthmatic children through substituting professional houseparents for the patient's own parents during an experimental two-week period while each child actually remained at home. Clearly, therefore, therapeutic intervention may be pursued through a variety of devices for environmental manipulation.

5. **The purveyors of intervention**
Finally, there is the controversial issue of who best conducts treatment. At one extreme, there are arguments in favour of 'the continuous reassuring support of the paediatrician (as essential) for the emotional and social adaptation of the young bleeder' (Mattsson and Gross, 1966). In adolescent haemophilia, the doctor assumes the extra mantle of a 'strong authoritative but accepting father figure' (Spencer and Behar, 1969). Battle (1972) sees him as professional ombudsman 'interpreting, integrating, and implementing the total care.'

It may be that in anxiety-provoking problems such as haemophilia, or in Battle's illustration of cranio-facial congenital malformation involving a complex of specialties, there is particular need for paediatric oversight because of the medical 'flavour' of treatment, or the relative rarity of the lesion. For example, 'The average general practitioner or paediatrician has not seen more than three or four blind youngsters in his practice . . . (nor has he had) much exposure to blindness in his medical training. (Hence) he has . . . little understanding of the complex problems and (is) . . . frequently . . . overly pessimistic or optimistic (in the advice he gives)' (Jan *et al.* 1973). Hence, the indication for the specialist's position as team coordinator in this instance.

Even so, the role is far from standard as confirmed by Blumenthal (1969) in recording viewpoints voiced by parents of retarded and fibrocystic children. In this study, a composite picture clearly emerges of the 'most helpful' and 'least helpful' physician as conceived by the 'consumer.'

Starfield and Borkowf (1969) make the point that traditionally, physicians are more alerted to somatic presentations than to behaviourally couched complaints, *i.e.* they are not attuned to other than physical symptoms. Indeed, 'It may be considered that . . . social and educational problems are outside the medical field, but who other than the doctor is better placed to grasp their full implications?' (Holdaway, 1972). Better placed he may be, but as Holdaway goes on to say, 'Few of us are adequately trained in this sphere.'

Because 'this skill . . . is at present relatively infrequently found in the medical profession, where it still depends more on personality than on training,' Lowit (1973) argues that 'the major resource to meet the needs of (the crisis created by chronic illness in childhood) lies in social workers.' Supporting this argument, Margaret Richards (1969) lists a bewildering array of professional helpers, both in England and the United States, ostensibly at hand to offer assistance, but in practice so difficult to mobilize as to justify the coordinating role of medical social worker as a kind of 'team spokesman' to avoid at least some of the dangers of overlap and contradiction. Joan Morse (1966) herself a social worker, predictably echoes this theme. Perhaps McCollum and Gibson (1970) advocate the best compromise through the co-ordinated support programme they operate conjointly as medical social worker and paediatrician in the management of children with cystic fibrosis.

However, in planning intervention, sufficient evidence now exists about the overriding import of personality factors in the therapist (Truax and Carkhuff, 1967) to justify the trial of non-professional personnel in therapeutic roles. Indeed, one of us (IBP) has experimented extensively with non-professional 'family counsellors', to assist in the care of handicapped children (see p. 95). Over a five-year period, the results indicate that for many of the roles traditionally performed by social workers, such women, if selected with due attention to their personality attributes, may prove equally effective and even on occasion, more so (Pless and Satterwhite, 1975).

As Truax and Carkhuff conclude, in respect of therapeutic effectiveness, the personal characteristics of the therapist may be *more* important than his professional status or training.

In the last analysis, 'The crucial recommendation, without which everything else is . . . valueless, is . . . continuously available access to one person . . .' Whether, as Maddison and

Raphael suggest, he or she must be professionally trained, *e.g.* doctor or social worker, or whether in time, lesser degrees of training will prove equally efficacious and acceptable, is a question still to be answered.

EMERGENT PRINCIPLES

A formula for intervention

So far, this has been an exercise in analysis — of the relevant factors involved in intervention. Complementary to it is surely the need for synthesis; that is, to evolve a concerted plan of action. Whether aimed at primary, secondary or tertiary prevention, that plan, to be successful, must take cognisance of individual patterns of adjustment as we identify them in each case formulation. This means, according to the integrated model we proposed earlier (page 29), fostering better coping strategies and buttressing self-concepts otherwise in danger of faltering. The processes whereby these objects are achieved are three-fold: Education, Counselling and Practical Provision.

Education

In respect of the disease itself, education means providing information (briefing), explanation (rendering in lay terms) and instruction (training), with access when required to expert management and advice.

Information, explanation and instruction

Factual data about the disease should always be available to the parents, and to the child himself, in as much detail as they can comfortably absorb without feeling confused. Numerous studies confirm the limited extent to which parents are able to comprehend the basic details of their child's illness (Etzwiler, 1962; Karp *et al.*, 1970; Sibinga and Friedman, 1971; Pless *et al.*, 1974). Yet, although few experiments have been successful in attempting to relate the extent of knowledge to degree of success in management of the disease, Miller has reported that preventable admissions for diabetes mellitus fell from 50% to 28% in the year following the introduction of a teaching programme in Los Angeles. (Laron, 1970). In other words, briefing should be both comprehensible and as comprehensive as possible.

It must also be authoritative, to command confidence; completely frank to safeguard credibility; consistent, as between one consultation and another, or between one doctor and another, to avoid misunderstanding; and repeated as often as need be to ensure that it has registered.

Maxwell and Gane (1962) epitomize these principles in their comments about the impact of congenital heart disease on the child's family: 'What does an average family know about congenital heart disease? A lot? A little? Do people really understand what doctors talk about? Do doctors help families in adjusting — whatever 'adjusting' means?' . . . 'The study suggests that emotional or other reasons may prevent the full impact of the explanation. Therefore, repeat it, and beware of the small percentage who cannot accept the possibility that their child has heart disease.' '. . . Fear and its variants are widespread in the family . . . (since) comprehensible explanation drives out fear . . . this was the usual basis for the leading role of the physician in helping the family to adjust.'

The need for clarity is reiterated by other workers in this field, *e.g.* Battle (1972), Mattsson (1972). There are so many imponderables unavoidably associated with individual chronic illnesses in childhood that additional ambiguity is to be avoided at all costs. Meadow (1969), in her study of congenital deafness, refers to the ambiguities inherent in the nature of the disorder and demonstrates how parental responses to them 'often determines the immediate and long-term course of the deaf child's adaptation to auditory deprivation.'

The more effective the briefing, therefore, in all these various aspects, the less the danger of persisting misconceptions and continuing prejudice. A balance must be struck however between relieving anxiety through clearing up false impressions, and generating fresh fear through half understood explanations.

This introduces the element of *timing*, a critical factor already referred to (page 190) in respect of ensuring optimum impact. Even so, great tolerance is called for in reviewing the problem, again and again, using different words perhaps to reinforce the point (Kennell *et al.* 1969).

Access to technical expertise
In an average paediatric practice of some two thousand children, years may pass before a case is encountered of (say) haemophilia, cystic fibrosis, diabetes or phenylketonuria. Many of these chronic childhood illnesses in fact are so relatively uncommon that the average doctor's experience of any given disorder will be correspondingly limited — a point emphasized by Jan *et al.* (1973) in relation to blind children.

But being conscious nevertheless of his overall responsibility, the primary physician (general practitioner or paediatrician) may well feel the need on occasion to seek the advice of a specialist colleague better versed in the particular problem. The prerogative should be his to consult with that expert, without in any way undermining the family's confidence in him — indeed only with their explicit approval. There is comfort in the knowledge, both for parents and for the physician, that where necessary, the best available technical resources have been mobilized to meet the immediate threat. Thereby, at least one major source of anxiety can be curtailed which would otherwise affect the child.

But not all specialists are alike. They differ markedly in temperament and technique of approach. Yet it is the family who will be 'exposed' to this encounter, not the referring doctor. Hence, part of the primary practitioner's skill lies in the art of selecting the 'right' specialist for the family in question. Experience will teach him which expert to 'marry' with which particular case, depending on their respective characteristics.

Primary responsibility, therefore, extends to deciding *when* expert opinion is called for, *where* best to mobilize it from the available resources in the area, and *whose* opinion it should be.

One more facet of the physician's judgment is called into play in this composite exercise. He must also decide when *not* to implement the specialized treatment recommended, or at least to what extent it should be modified. For example, the consultant neurologist may recommend a schedule of anticonvulsants for the epileptic child which, while successfully controlling seizures, also curtails the patient's level of academic performance in school. If failure in scholastic achievement represents a potential source of tension for the gifted older child, or important examinations are at stake, the family doctor armed with this more intimate knowledge, may well advise reducing medication even at the risk of the occasional seizure supervening. In this decision, he should carry the parents unequivocally with him.

Counselling
Judgments of this kind, embodying the very art of medicine, can only be made by doctors who are both interested and competent in the management of the child as a person, over and above their competence in treating the illness. In other words, technical expertise is not synonymous with expert management of the patient.

This is a fresh dimension, calling for knowledge in depth of both the child and his family. To achieve it demands time, energy and skill, an investment which not all doctors endorse as lying within the orbit of their professional responsibility. Some take the view that the business of medicine is purely to attend to organic disease. Others regard the care of chronic illness as more properly the purview of the systems specialist. Others again prefer the role of team coordinator, deputing field work to paramedical personnel as and where these are available in the community.

Irrespective of the doctor's personal philosophy, however, there can be no doubt that the key to successful treatment in depth is a positive relationship of confidence and trust between the doctor, the patient and his family (Korsch *et al.*, 1968). Even the imparting of medical information has been shown to be affected by this basic relationship (Sibinga and Friedman, 1971) in that neither timing nor adequacy of data alone is sufficient to achieve a satisfactory level of understanding. Nor is this simply a function of the parents' intelligence. For example, Keleske *et al.* (1967), studying parental reactions to phenylketonuria, conclude that: 'Efforts to impose dietary restriction . . . affect the emotional climate of the total family; (such) that the parents need constant support, orientation and counselling to enable them to maintain a realistic attitude . . .'

What does this relationship entail? It involves sharing the experience with the child and with his parents, permitting them the opportunity to ask questions, to check perplexing details, and to ventilate anxieties about the nature of the illness, the significance of treatment, and the uncertainties of prognosis.

To induce the requisite aura for this development, requires the projection of a tolerant, uncritical and personally involved professional image which cannot be engendered unless genuinely felt.

Essentially, this is the art of counselling, embodying, as it does, encouragement and support, the strengthening of emotional resources, and the implication of 'being with' the patient and his family, rather than 'doing things to' them (Wolff, 1971). The secret of its achievement is to forego the tradition of 'talking to' the patient, *i.e.* didactic therapeutic instruction, in favour of *listening* as the problem unfolds, and listening with *empathy*.

In other words, education is a two-way process, *i.e.* not only from doctor to patient by way of providing medical information, but equally from patient to doctor, by way of therapeutic feedback, so that he can better gauge each family's level of tolerance and optimum philosophy for coping.

Training in communication

To achieve this more subtle level of intervention involves 'teaching (paediatric trainees) how to recognize and deal with family situations in which emotional problems aggravate chronic illness' (Russack and Friedman, 1970). This is by no means a novel recommendation. The same plea was made by Korsch and her associates twenty years ago (1954). Yet fifteen years later, their reference to 'gaps in doctor-patient communication' remains as apposite as ever (Korsch *et al.*, 1968) — eloquent testimony to continuing resistance to any innovation in medical education.

The need to teach psychotherapeutic skills to medical students in respect of parent counselling, is repeatedly referred to in recent literature. Recognizing the dangers of emotional sensitivity among uninitiated medical counsellors. Woodmansey (1971) wisely recommends screening procedures to overcome any such natural 'Achilles' heel.'

Just as many problems may arise, however, from the converse situation of emotional insensitivity. 'The complexity of human personality is such that casual observation by an untrained or insensitive observer tells us virtually nothing,' *e.g.* 'in one study of children with rheumatic fever and their mothers . . . many of the really relevant anxieties . . . did not emerge until (after) ten to fifteen interviews'.

'Doctors . . . are prone to interpret passive conformity and 'good behaviour' as evidence that things are going well and that no psychological sequelae are to be anticipated . . . (yet) shutting one's eyes to psychological complexities does not make them go away.' (Maddison and Raphael, 1971).

A further paradox in this field is that 'in chronic disability it is often the patient and his family who . . . have a better knowledge of the disease, . . . (its) treatment and . . . implications . . . than do the health personnel . . . In short, it is they, and not the doctors or nurses, who become the experts.' (Davis, 1974).

In these circumstances, demonstrating the advantages of doctor-patient communication becomes doubly difficult, especially when set against the more familiar role of the traditional medical model.

Continuity of relationship

Obstacles of this kind notwithstanding, assuming a change in medical school curricula sufficient to foster enhanced communication skills, the further factor necessary to consolidate such expertise is *continuity of contact.* Nothing is more calculated to undermine confidence and add to the confusion than fragmentation of professional contact. 'We saw a different doctor each time and they did not seem to know what we had been told' is hardly likely to inspire parental trust. In the current climate of shared responsibility within primary practitioner partnerships, community health care teams, or medical 'firms' in hospital, conflict of opinion is a potential danger arising from discontinuity. If, however, the professional group retains its cohesion as an operational team, the element of constancy may be sufficiently safeguarded to satisfy most parents even though certain members may come and go. Indeed, a minor degree of 'turnover' among key members may actually be beneficial through rekindling of interest periodically. Provided that continuity is preserved in the sense of an 'institutional memory', there may be more to be gained than having the same physician all the time, if, through non-involvement, he is unable to recall what has gone before.

While in no sense underrating the prime significance of a sustained relationship without which '(the mother) is unable to ventilate the anxieties, guilts and resentments which, repressed, or suppressed, within her, will complicate the handling of her sick child' (Maddison and Raphael, 1971), there is nevertheless cold comfort in counselling alone. These families need succour as well as support.

Practical provision
Traditionally, it is the primary physician who is most favourably placed to assess priorities for the family in need and translate them into action. To what extent he personally intervenes depends upon the problem, the resources available, the accessibility of allied personnel, and of course the individual doctor. But what he can and *should* be prepared to do, irrespective of his professional ethos, is to act as catalyst, *i.e.* to mobilize or activate such services or facilities as may be required. The first prerequisite of any health care system is its delivery. If this sounds self-evident or trite, consider Helsel's comments (1967) about long-term care — 'even in communities where many of the elements of long-term care are available, services are fragmented and not organized into a functioning pattern providing a continuum of care.' Numerous recent reports (*e.g.* Carnegie U.K. Trust, Living with Handicap; The Rand study by Brewer and Kakalik) each provide abundant evidence for this assertion.

The doctor then represents a bridge, so to speak, between his handicapped patients and their families, and the care provisions locally available, to ensure that the 'consumers' actually get to them. At one end of the spectrum, the facility may be circumscribed — the orthopaedic appliance, the specialized, transport, the pre-school nursery enrolment, the home-visiting contact, the neighbourhood counselling service. At the other end, a much more comprehensive approach is called for, best exemplified perhaps by the needs of the child with multiple handicaps.

Referring for example to evaluation of the multi-handicapped blind child, Jan *et al.* (1973) firmly stipulate that 'it is not possible to determine the individual's potential unless the full extent of his handicaps, detailed social information, and the degree and quality of stimulation to which he has been exposed, are known. There is a need, therefore, for a multi-disciplinary team approach to the evaluation and treatment of blind children. Such a team should include . . . teachers of the blind . . . psychologists, medical and other health personnel . . . (with) special knowledge of the developmental peculiarities of these children.'

Bleck and Headley (1961), referring much earlier to the value of a multi-disciplined approach to the problems of cerebral palsied children, claim that it eliminates 'not only . . . financial waste, but emotional waste as well.' In England, this trend has been reflected in the relatively recent introduction of assessment centres for the investigation and management of multiply-handicapped children, organized either by the neighbourhood local authority, or by the regional children's hospital (*British Medical Journal* Leader, 1971; Department of Education and Science Publication, 1971).

A note of caution, however, is sounded by Battle (1972). 'While admirable in concept, the (multi-disciplinary) approach has not in itself resulted in optimal care. Instead, fragmented care and lack of integration . . . have often produced a poorly conceived medical programme . . .' Sometimes, the very multiplicity of personnel, 'approximately thirty persons for each handicapped child', may defeat its own purpose by generating confusion and incoordination.

The ideal linkage, it would seem, is between the technical expertise and investigational facilities of the hospital-based service and the rehabilitative potential of the community-based service, with the family doctor acting as entrepreneur between the two.

His own role, to summarize, is the composite one of educator, counsellor and action catalyst, in the pursuit of successful intervention.

Conclusion
In the final analysis, the key to these endeavours is *care* — or rather, more precisely, *caring*; not necessarily the *amount* of care as measured in unit time (as shown by Perrin *et al.,* 1972); nor for that matter, its comprehensive character, since multiplicity of disciplines can just as readily cause confusion; nor indeed in 'concrete' terms of cure, correction or reduction of morbidity, in the sense defined by Lewis (1971), although these certainly lend themselves to objective measurement; but in the more intangible sense of *quality* of care, which, if not individually perpetuated, should at least be both persistent and personalized. This is a difficult property to define, though easier perhaps to recognize in those who practise it. It is reflected in the attitude which prompts us to include, in our approach to parents, the simple reassurance that their feelings are 'perfectly normal and biologically natural'. (Battle) — elementary perhaps, but revealing nevertheless in its humanity.

As Peabody (1927) has so eloquently expressed it: 'The secret of care of the patient lies in caring *for* the patient.'

References

ABERCROMBIE, M. L. J. and TYSON, M. C. (1966). Body image and draw-a-man test in cerebral palsy. *Developmental Medicine and Child Neurology*, **8**, 9.

ACK, M., MILLER, I. and WEIL, W. B., Jr. (1961). Intelligence of children with diabetes mellitus. *Pediatrics*, **28**, 764.

AGLE, D. P. (1964). Psychiatric studies of patients with hemophilia and related states. *Archives of Internal Medicine*, **114**, 76.

AGLE, D. P. and MATTSSON, A. (1968). Psychiatric and social care of patients with hereditary hemorrhagic disease. *Modern Treatment*, **5**, 11.

AISENBERG, R. B., WOLFF, P. H., ROSENTHAL, M. A. and NADAS, A. S. (1973). Psychological impact of cardiac catheterization. *Pediatrics*, **51**, 1051.

ALBERMAN, E. D., BUTLER, N. and GARDINER, P. A. (1971). Children with squints. A handicapped group? *Practitioner*, **206**, 501.

ALEXANDER, A. B., MIKLICH, D. R. and HERSHKOFF, H. (1972). The immediate effects of systematic relaxation training on peak expiratory flow rates in asthmatic children. *Psychosomatic Medicine*, **XXXIV**, 388.

ALLEN, F. H. and PEARSON, G. H. J. (1928). The emotional problems of the physically handicapped child. *British Journal of Medical Psychology*, **8**, 212.

ALLEN, G. H. (1967). Aspirations and expectations of physically impaired high school seniors. *Personnel and Guidance Journal*, **47**, 59.

ANDERSON, E. M. (1974). *The Disabled Schoolchild: A Study of Integration in Primary Schools*. Methuen, London.

APLEY, J., BARBOUR, R. F. and WESTMACOTT, I. (1967). Impact of congenital heart disease on the family: Preliminary report. *British Medical Journal*, **1**, 103.

BADELL-RIBERA, A., SCHULMAN, K. and PADDOCK, N. (1966). The relationship of non-progressive hydrocephalus to intellectual functioning in children with spina bifida cystica. *Pediatrics*, **37**, 787.

BAGLEY, C. (1971). *The Social Psychology of the Epileptic Child*. University of Miami Press, Coral Gables, Florida.

BARCAI, A. (1970). Emotional factors and control in juvenile diabetes. In *Habilitation and Rehabilitation of Juvenile Diabetes. Proceedings of First Beilinson Symposium on Juvenile Diabetes.* p. 108 (Z. T. Laron, ed.). Williams & Wilkins, Baltimore.

BARKER, R. G., WRIGHT, B. A., MYERSON, L. and GONICK, M. R. (1953). *Adjustment to Physical Handicap and Illness: A Survey of the Social Psychology of Physique and Disability.* Social Science Research Council (Revised), New York.

BARNES, C. M., KENNY, F. M., CAWL, T. and REINHART, J. B. (1972). Measurement in management of anxiety in children for open heart surgery. *Pediatrics,* 49, 250.

BARSCH, R. H. (1968). *The Parent of the Handicapped Child.* Thomas, Springfield, Illinois.

BATTLE, C. U. (1972). The role of the pediatrician as ombudsman in the health care of the young handicapped child. *Pediatrics,* 50, 1916.

BATTLE, C. U. (1974). Disruptions in the socialization of a young, severely handicapped child. *Rehabilitation Literature,* 35, 130.

BAUS, G. J., LETSON, L. L. and RUSSELL, E. (1958). Group session for parents of children with epilepsy. *Journal of Pediatrics,* 52, 270.

BELLAK, L. and BELLAK, S. S. (1955). *The Children's Apperception Tests, 1952-1955. CAT Supplement.* Scribner, New York.

BENDER, L. and FARETRA, G. (1963). Body Image Problems of Children. In *Psychological Basis of Medical Practice.* p. 431. (Liev, H., Lief, V., Lief, N., eds.). Harper and Row, New York.

BENTOVIM, A. (1972a). Emotional disturbances of handicapped pre-school children and their families—attitudes to the child. *British Medical Journal,* 3, 579.

BENTOVIM, A. (1972b). Handicapped pre-school children and their families—effect on child's emotional development. *British Medical Journal,* 3, 634.

BERGGREEN, S. M. (1971). A study of the mental health of the near relatives of 20 multihandicapped children. *Acta Paediatrica Scandinavica,* Supplement 215.

BERGMAN, A. B. and STAMM, S. J. (1967). The morbidity of cardiac nondisease in schoolchildren. *New England Journal of Medicine,* 276, 1008.

BERK, R. L. (1963). The psychological impact of contact lenses on children and youth. *Journal of the American Optometric Association,* 34, 1217.

BERNSTEIN, I. L., ALLEN, J. E., KREINDLER, L., GHORY, J. E. and WOHL, T. H. (1960). A community approach to juvenile intractable asthma. *Pediatrics,* 26, 586.

BLECK, E. E. and HEADLEY, L. (1961). Treatment and parent

counselling for the pre-school child with cerebral palsy. *Pediatrics*, **27**, 1026.

BLOM, G. E. and Nicholls, G. (1954). Emotional factors in children with rheumatoid arthritis. *American Journal of Orthopsychiatry*, **24**, 588.

BLUMENTHAL, M. (1969). Experiences of parents of retardates and children with cystic fibrosis. *Archives of General Psychiatry*, **21**, 160.

BOBROVE, P. (1964). *Adjustment to auditory disability in adolescents*. Doctoral Dissertation, University of Rochester, Rochester, New York.

BOOTH, B. P. (1965). Residential courses for families with a handicapped child — an experiment. *Case Conference*, 60.

BOWER, E. M. (1960). *Early Identification of Emotionally Handicapped Children in School*. Thomas, Springfield, Illinois.

BOWER, E. and LAMBERT, N. (1962). *A Class Play*. California State Department of Education, Educational Testing Service, Princeton, New Jersey.

BOWLEY, A. H. (1967). A follow-up study of 64 children with cerebral palsy. *Developmental Medicine and Child Neurology*, **9**, 172.

BOWLEY, A. and GARDNER, L. (1972). *The Handicapped Child*. Churchill Livingstone, Edinburgh.

BREWER, G. C. and KAKALIK, J, S. (1974). *Improving services to handicapped children: Summary and recommendations*. (Prepared for the Department of HEW. Office of the Assistant Secretary for Planning and Evaluation). The Rand Corp., Santa Monica, Calif.

BRIELAND, D. (1967). A follow up study of orthopedically handicapped high school graduates. *Exceptional Children*, **33**, 555.

BROIDA, D. C., IZARD, C. E. and CRUICKSHANK, W. M. (1950). Thematic apperception reaction of crippled children. *Journal of Clinical Psychology*, **3**, 243.

BRONFENBRENNER, U. (1970). Some reflections on 'antecedents of optimal psychology adjustment'. *Journal of Consulting and Clinical Psychology*, **35**, 296.

BRONKS, I. G. and BLACKBURN, E. K. (1968). A socio-medical study of haemophilia and related states. *British Journal of Preventive and Social Medicine*, **22**, 68.

BROWN, F. (1934). A psychoneurotic inventory for children between nine and fourteen years of age. *Journal of Applied Psychology*, **18**, 566.

BROWNE, W. J., MALLY, M. A. and KANE, R. P. (1960). Psychological aspects of hemophilia: a study of twenty-eight hemophilic children and their families. *American Journal of Orthopsychiatry*, **30**, 730.

BRUHN, J. G., HAMPTON, J. W. and CHANDLER, B. C. (1970). Clinical

marginality and psychological adjustment in hemophilia. *Journal of Psychosomatic Research*, **15**, 207.
BRYT, A. (1966). Psychiatric considerations in candidates for plastic surgery, *Eye, Ear, Nose and Throat Monthly*, **45**, 102.
BUCK, J. N. (1948). House-Tree-Person. The H-T-P Technique: A Qualitative and Quantitative Scoring Manual. *Journal of Clinical Psychology*, Monograph Supplement 5, 1.
BURLINGHAM, D. (1961). Some notes on the development of the blind. *Psychoanalytic Study of the Child*, **16**, 121.
BUROS, E. (1972). *Mental Measurements Handbook*, 7th ed. Gryphon Press, New Jersey.
BUROS, E. (1970). *Personality Tests and Reviews: Including an Index to the Mental Measurement Yearbooks*. Gryphon Press, New Jersey.
CANNING, H. and MAYER, J. (1966). Obesity—its possible effect on college acceptance. *New England Journal of Medicine*, **275**, 21.
CAPPON, D. and BANKS, R. (1968). Distorted body perception in obesity. *Journal of Nervous and Mental Disease*, **146**, 465.
CARLSEN, A. H. (1957). Vocational and social adjustment of physically handicapped students. *Exceptional Children*, **23**, 367.
CARLSON, R. (1970). On the structure of self-esteem: comments on Ziller's formulation. *Journal of Consulting and Clinical Psychology*, **34**, 264.
CARNEGIE UNITED KINGDOM TRUST (1964). *Handicapped Children and Their Families*. Constable, Edinburgh.
CASTANEDA, A., McCANDLESS, B. R. and PALERMO, D. S. (1956). The children's form of the Manifest Anxiety Scale. *Child Development*, **27**, 317.
CATTELL, R. B. and BICE, G. F. (1962). The Institute for Personality and Ability Testing, Champaign, Illinois.
CENTERS, L. and CENTERS, R. A. (1963a). A comparison of the body images of amputee and non-amputee children as revealed in figure drawings. *Journal of Projective Techniques and Personality Assessment*, **27**, 158.
CENTERS, L. and CENTERS, R. A. (1963b). Peer group attitudes toward the amputee child. *Journal of Social Psychology*, **61**, 127.
CLEVELAND, S., REITMAN, E. and BREWER, E. (1965). Psychological factors in juvenile rheumatoid arthritis. *Arthritis and Rheumatism*, **8**, 1152.
CLIFFORD, E. (1965). Connotative meaning of self- and asthma-related concepts for two subgroups of asthmatic children. *Journal of Psychology*, **8**, 467.
CLIFFORD, E. (1969). The impact of symptom: a preliminary comparison of clift lip-palate and asthmatic children. *Cleft Palate*

Journal, **6**, 221.
COHEN, J. (1966). The effects of blindness on children. *Children*, **13**, 23.
COLLIER, B. N. (1969a). Comparison between adolescents with and without diabetes. *Personnel and Guidance Journal*, **49**, 679.
COLLIER, B. N. (1969b). Interpersonal traits of secondary school adolescents with or without diabetes. *Rehabilitation Counselling Bulletin*, Dec., 190.
COLLIER, B. N., Jr. and ETZWILER, D. (1971). Comparative study of diabetes knowledge among juvenile diabetics and their parents. *Diabetes*, **20**, 51.
COLVIN, R. W. (1964). *Self Concept as a Research Dimension in Mental Retardation: the Presentation of a Rationale and a Method (The Silhouette Test of Self Concept and Interpersonal Relations).* p. 1. American Association on Mental Deficiency, Kansas City, Missouri.
CONVERSE, J. M. and ROGERS, B. O. (1963). *Conference on Facial Disfigurement: A Rehabilitation Problem.* US Department of Health, Education and Welfare, Vocational Rehabilitation Administration, Washington, DC.
COOPERSMITH, S. (1959). A method of determining types of self esteem. *Journal of Abnormal and Social Psychology*, **59**, 87.
COURT, S. D. M. (1971). Child health in a changing community. *British Medical Journal*, **2**, 125.
COWEN, E. L., UNDERBERG, R. P., VERRILLO, R. T. and BENHAM, F. G. (1961). *Adjustment to Visual Disability in Adolescence.* American Foundation for the Blind, New York.
COWEN, E. L., HUSER, J., BEACH, D. R. and RAPPAPORT, J. (1970). Parental perceptions of young children and their relation to indexes of adjustment. *Journal of Consulting and Clinical Psychology*, **34**, 97.
COWEN, E. L., PEDERSON, A., BABIGIAN, H., IZZO, L. D. and TROST, M. A. (1973). Long-term follow-up of early detected vulnerable children. *Journal of Consulting and Clinical Psychology*, **41**, 438.
COWIE, V. (1967). Parental counselling and spina bifida. *Developmental Medicine and Child Neurology*, **9**, 110.
CRAIN, A. J., SUSSMAN, M. B. and WEIL, W. B., Jr. (1966). Effects of a diabetic child on marital integration and related measures of family functioning. *Journal of Health and Human Behavior*, **7**, 122.
CREAK, M. (1971). Gaps in medical education. *Proceedings of the Royal Society of Medicine*, **65**, 106.
CREER, T. L. (1970). The use of a time-out from positive reinforcement procedure with asthmatic children. *Journal of Psycho-*

somatic Research, 14, 117.
CREER, T. L. and YOCHES, C. (1971). The modification of an inappropriate behavioural pattern in asthmatic children. *Journal of Chronic Diseases*, 24, 507.
CROTHERS, B. and PAINE, R. S. (1959). *The Natural History of Cerebral Palsy*. Oxford University Press, London.
CROWTHER, D. L. (1967). Psychosocial aspects of epilepsy. *Pediatric Clinics of North America*, 14, 921.
CRUICKSHANK, W. M. (1952). A study of the relation of physical disability to social adjustment. *American Journal of Occupational Therapy*, 1, 100.
CRUICKSHANK, W. M. (1963). *Psychology of Exceptional Children and Youth*. Prentice-Hall, Englewood Cliffs, New Jersey.
CUMMINGS, S. L., BAYLEY, H. C. and RIE, H. E. (1966). Effect of the child's deficiency on the mother: A study of mothers of mentally retarded, chronically ill and neurotic children. *American Journal of Orthopsychiatry*, 36, 595.
DALTON, K. (1968). Menstruation and examinations. *Lancet*, 4, 1386.
DAVIE, R., BUTLER, N. and GOLDSTEIN, H. (1972). *From Birth to Seven: A Report of the National Child Development Study*. Longman, London.
DAVIS, F. (1961). Deviance disavowal: The management of strained interaction by the visibly handicapped. *Social Problems*, 9, 1.
DAVIS, F. (1963). *Passage Through Crisis. Polio Victims and Their Families*. Bobbs-Merrill, Indianapolis, Ind.
DAVIS, F. (1974). *The Chronically Disabled and The Family, Present Predicaments and Some Future Prospects*. Minnesota Family Study Center Graduate Symposium on Health and the Family. University of Minnesota, Minneapolis, Minnesota. (Unpublished.)
DEBUSKY, M. and DOMBRO, R. H. (1970). *The Chronically Ill Child and His Family*. Thomas, Springfield, Illinois.
DEFRIES, Z. and BROWDER, S. (1952). Group therapy with epileptic children and their mothers. *Bulletin of the New York Academy of Medicine*, 28, 235.
DEMB, N. and RUESS, A. L. (1967). High school drop-out rate for cleft palate patients. *Cleft Palate Journal*, 4, 327.
DEMBO, T., LADIEU, G. and WRIGHT, B. (1948). *Adjustment to Misfortune: A Study in Social-Emotional Relationships Between Injured and Non-injured People*. Final Report to the Army Medical Research & Development Board, Office of the Surgeon General, War Department, Washington, DC.
DEMBO, T., LEVITON, G. L. and WRIGHT, B. A. (1956). Adjustment to misfortune — a problem of social psychological rehabilitation.

Artificial Limbs, **3**, 4.
DENSEN, P. M., ULLMAN, D. B., JONES, E. W. and VANDOW, J. (1970). Childhood characteristics as indicators of adult health status. *Public Health Reports*, **85**, 981.
DESCHIN, C. S. and NASH, M. V. (1971). *Children Together—The Effect of Integrated Group Experiences on Orthopedically Handicapped Children*. A Final Report to the National Institute of Mental Health for Research, Washington, DC.
DIBNER, A. S. and DIBNER, S. S. (1971). Integration or segregation of deviants? The physically handicapped child. *Community Mental Health Journal*, **7**, 227.
DINNAGE, R. (1970). *The Handicapped Child. Studies in Child Development Research Review, Vol. I*. Longman, London.
DINNAGE, R. (1972). *The Handicapped Child. Studies in Child Development Research Review, Vol. II*. Longman, London.
DOLL, E. A. (1965). *Vineland Social Maturity Scale*. American Guidance Service, Inc., Circle Pines, Minnesota.
DORNER, S. (1973). Psychological and social problems of families of adolescent spina bifida patients: a preliminary report. *Developmental Medicine and Child Neurology*, **15**, Supplement 29, 24.
DORNER, S. and ELTON, A. (1973). Short, taught and vulnerable. *Special Education*, **62**, 12.
DOUGLAS, J. W. B., ROSS, J. M. and SIMPSON, H. R. (1967). The ability and attainment of short-sighted pupils. *Journal of the Royal Statistical Society. Series A (General)*, **130**, 479.
DOUGLAS, J. W. B., ROSS, J. M. and SIMPSON, H. R. (1968). *All Our Future—A Longitudinal Study of Secondary Education*. Davies, London.
DOWLING, J. P. (1960). Preventing dependency patterns in chronically ill children. *Social Casework*, **XLI**, 395.
DOWNEY, J. A. and LOW, N. L. (1974). *The Child With Disabling Illness: Principles of Rehabilitation*. Saunders, Philadelphia, Penna.
DOWNING, R. W., MOED, G. and WRIGHT, B. W. (1961). Studies of disability: A technique for psychological measurement of effects. *Child Development*, **32**, 561.
DUBO, S., McLEAN, J. A., CHING, A. Y. T., WRIGHT, H. L., KAUFFMAN, P. E. and SHELDON, J. (1961). A study of relationships between family situation, bronchial asthma and personal adjustment in children. *Journal of Pediatrics*, **59**, 402.
DUNSDON, M. G. (1952). *The Educability of Cerebral Palsy Children*. Newnes, London.
EASSON, W. M. (1966). Psychopathological environmental reaction to congenital defect. *Journal of Nervous and Mental Disease*, **142**,

453.
EPILEPSY FOUNDATION (1967). *Summaries of Articles on Juvenile Epilepsy.* Epilepsy Foundation, Washington, DC.
ETZWILER, D. D. (1962). What the juvenile diabetic knows about his disease. *Pediatrics,* **29,** 135.
EYSENCK, H. J. (1959). *Manual of the Maudsley Personality Inventory.* University of London Press, London.
EYSENCK, H. J. (1965). The Rorschach. In *Mental Measurements Year Book* (Buros, O.K., ed.). University of London Press, London.
EYSENCK, S. B. G. (1965). A new scale for personality measurement in children. *British Journal of Educational Psychology,* **XXXV**, 362.
FARBER, B. (1959). Effects of a severely mentally retarded child on family integration. *Society for Research in Child Development,* **24,** 2.
FEINBERG, T., LATTIMER, J. K., JETER, K., LANGFORD, W. and BECK, L. (1974). Questions that worry children with exstrophy. *Pediatrics,* **53,** 242.
FEINSTEIN, A. R., TAUBE, H., CAVALIERI, R., SCHULTZ, S. C. and KRYLE, L. (1962). Physical activities and rheumatic heart disease in asymptomatic patients. *Journal of the American Medical Association,* **180,** 1028.
FELDT, R. H., EWERT, J. C., STICKLER, G. B. and WEIDMAN, W. H. (1969). Children with congenital heart disease. *American Journal of Diseases of Children,* **117,** 281.
FISHER, S. and CLEVELAND, S. E. (1958). *Body Image and Personality.* Von Nostrand, Princeton, New Jersey.
FITZIMMONS, R. (1958). Developmental, psychosocial and educational factors in non-organic articulation problems. *Child Development,* **29,** 486.
FLOYER, E. B. (1955). *A Psychological Study of a City's Cerebral Palsied Children.* British Council for the Welfare of Spastics, London.
FORCE, D. G., Jr. (1956). Social status of physically handicapped children. *Exceptional Children,* **23,** 104.
FOX, C., DAVIDSON, K., LIGHTHALL, F., WAITE, R. and SARASON, S. B. (1958). Human figure drawings of high and low anxious children. *Child Development,* **29,** 297.
FRANCIS-WILLIAMS, J. (1965). *Assessment of Cerebral Palsy Children. A Survey of Advances Since 1958.* National Association for Mental Health, London.
FRANKEL, J. J. (1970). Academic Performance of Juvenile Diabetics and Teachers' Attitudes. In *Habilitation and Rehabilitation of Juvenile Diabetics. Proceedings of First Beilinson Symposium on Juvenile Diabetes.* (Z. T. Laron, ed.), p. 93. Williams & Wilkins,

Baltimore.
FREEMAN, R. D. (1970). Psychiatric problems in adolescents with cerebral palsy. *Developmental Medicine and Child Neurology*, **12**, 64.
FREESTON, B. M. (1971). An enquiry into the effect of a spina bifida child upon family life. *Developmental Medicine and Child Neurology*, **13**, 456.
FREUD, A. (1946). *The Ego and the Mechanisms of Defence*. International University Press, New York.
FREUD, A. (1952). The role of bodily illness in the mental life of children. *Psychoanalytic Study of the Child*, **7**, 69.
GARDINER, A.. PORTEOUS, N. and WALTER-SMITH, J. H. (1972). The effect of coeliac disease on the mother-child relationship. *Australian Paediatric Journal*, **8**, 39.
GARDNER, W. I. (1967). Use of the California test of personality with the mentally retarded. *Mental Retardation*, **5**, 12.
GARLINGHOUSE, J. and SHARP, L. J. (1968). The hemophilic child's self-concept and family stress in relation to bleeding episodes. *Nursing Research*, **17**, 32.
GARRARD, S. D. and RICHMOND, J. B. (1963). Psychological aspects of the management of chronic diseases and handicapping conditions in childhood. In *The Psychological Basis of Medical Practice*, p. 307–403, (Lief, H., Lief, V., Lief, N. eds.). Harper & Row, New York.
GATES, M. F. (1946). A comparative study of some problems of social and emotional adjustment of crippled and non-crippled girls and boys. *Journal of Genetic Psychology*, **68**, 219.
GATH, A. (1973). The school-age siblings of mongol children. *British Journal of Psychiatry*, **123**, 161.
GATH, A. (1974). Sibling reactions to mental handicap: A comparison of the brothers and sisters of mongol children. *Journal of Child Psychology & Psychiatry*, **15**, 187.
GAYTON, W. F. and FRIEDMAN, S. (1973). Psychosocial aspects of cystic fibrosis. *American Journal of Diseases of Children*, **126**, 856.
GEIGER, A., BARTA, L. and HUBAY, M. (1973). Diabetes and mental state. *Acta Paediatrica Academiae Scientiarum Hungaricae*, **14**, 119.
GLASER, H. H., HARRISON, G. S. and LYNN, D. B. (1964). Emotional implications of congenital heart disease in children. *Pediatrics*, **33**, 367.
GLASER, H. H., LYNN, D. B. and HARRISON, G. S. (1961). Comprehensive medical care for handicapped children. *American Journal of Diseases of Children*, **102**, 344.

GLASNER, P. J. (1949). Personality characteristics and emotional problems in stutterers under the age of five. *Journal of Speech and Hearing Disorders,* **14**, 135.

GLUCKSMAN, M. L. and HIRSCH, J. (1969). The response of obese patients to weight reduction. *Psychosomatic Medicine,* **XXXI**, 1.

GOETZINGER, C. P., HARRISON, C. and BAER, C. J. (1964). Small perceptive hearing loss: Its effect in school-age children. *Volta Review,* **66**, 124.

GOETZINGER, C. P., ORTIZ, J. D., BELLEROSE, B. and BUCHAN, L. G. (1966). A study of the S. O. Rorschach with deaf and hearing adolescents. *American Annals of the Deaf,* **111**, 510.

GOETZINGER, C. P. and PROUD, G. O. (1966). *Severe Early Deafness; Its Effect Upon an Individual's Mental and Emotional Well-being.* Department of Otorhinolaryngology and Hearing and Speech, University of Kansas School of Medicine, Salina, Kansas.

GOLDBERG, R. and SATOW, K. (1972). Vocational development of adults with congenital heart disease. *Rehabilitation Psychology,* **19**, 4.

GOLDIE, L. (1966). The psychiatry of the handicapped family. *Developmental Medicine and Child Neurology,* **8**, 456.

GOLDIN, G. J., PERRY, S. L., MARGOLIN, R. J., STOTSKY, B. A. and FOSTER, J. C. (1971). *The Rehabilitation of the Young Epileptic.* Heath, Lexington, Mass.

GOUGH, H. G. and HEILBRUN, A. B. (1965). *Adjective Check List Manual.* Consulting Psychologists Press, Palo Alto, California.

GRAHAM, P. and RUTTER, M. (1970). Psychiatric aspects of physical disorder. In *Education, Health and Behaviour,* p. 309. (Rutter, M., Tizard, J. and Whitmore, K., eds.). Longman, London.

GRAHAM, P., RUTTER, M., YULE, W. and PLESS, I. B. (1967). Childhood asthma: a psychosomatic disorder? Some epidemiological considerations. *British Journal of Preventive and Social Medicine,* **21**, 78.

GRANTHAM, E. (1971). Handicapped children in pre-school playgroups. *British Medical Journal,* **4**, 346.

GREEN, J. B. and HARTLAGE, L. C. (1971). Comparative performance of epileptic and non-epileptic children and adolescents. *Diseases of the Nervous System,* **32**, 418.

GREEN, J. B. and HARTLAGE, L. C. (1972). The relation of parental attitudes to academic and social achievement in epileptic children. *Epilepsia,* **13**, 21.

GREEN, M. and DUROCHER, M. A. (1965). Improving parent care of handicapped children. *Children,* **12**, 185.

GREEN, M. and LEVITT, E. E. (1962). Constriction of body image in children with congenital heart disease. *Pediatrics,* **29**, 438.

GREEN, M. and SOLNIT, A. S. (1964). Reactions to the threatened loss of a child: A vulnerable child syndrome. *Pediatrics,* 34, 58.
GREIFER, I. and BARNETT, H. L. (1974). Maintenance hemodialysis and kidney transplantation in children — the role of the primary physician. *Pediatric Annals,* 3, 82.
GROKOEST, A., SNYDER, A. and SCHLEGER, R. (1962). *Juvenile Rheumatoid Arthritis.* Little, Brown, Boston.
GUNDERSON, E. K. E. (1965). Body size, self-evaluation and military effectiveness. *Journal of Personality and Social Psychology,* 2, 902.
GUNDERSON, E. K. E. and JOHNSON, L. C. (1965). Past experience, self evaluation, and present adjustment. *Journal of Social Psychology,* 66, 241.
GUNN, J. and FENTON, G. (1971). Epilepsy, automatism and crime. *Lancet,* 1, 1173.
HAHN, W. W. and CLARK, J. A. (1967). Psychophysiological reactivity of asthmatic children. *Psychosomatic Medicine,* **XXIX**, 526.
HANLON, T. E., HOFSTAETTER, P. R. and O'CONNOR, J. P. (1954). Congruence of self and ideal self in relation to personality adjustment. *Journal of Consulting Psychology,* 18, 215.
HARDY, R. E. (1968). A study of manifest anxiety among blind residential school students. *New Outlook for the Blind,* 48, 173.
HARRIS, D. B. (1961). *Measuring the Psychological Maturity of Children: A Revision and Extension of the Goodenough Draw-A-Man Test.* World Book, Tarrytown-on-Hudson, New York.
HARRIS, M. C. and SHURE, N. (1956). A study of behavior patterns in asthmatic children. *Journal of Allergy,* 27, 312.
HARROW, M., FOX, D. A., MARKHUS, K. L., STILLMAN, R. and HALLOWELL, C. B. (1968). Changes in adolescents' self-concepts and their parents' perceptions during psychiatric hospitalization. *Journal of Nervous and Mental Disease,* 147, 252.
HARWAY, V. T. (1962). Self evaluation and goal setting behavior in orthopedically handicapped children. In *Readings on the Exceptional Child,* p. 568. (Trapp, E. P. and Himmelstein, P. eds.). Methuen, London.
HELSEL, E. D. (1967). Planning ahead for long term care. *Developmental Medicine and Child Neurology,* 9, 757.
HERSOV, L. (1963). Emotional factors in cerebral palsy. *Developmental Medicine and Child Neurology,* 5, 504.
HESS, D. W. (1960). *The Evaluation of Personality and Adjustment in Deaf and Hearing Children Using a Nonverbal Modification of the Make A Picture Story (MAPS) Test.* Doctorate Thesis. University of Rochester, Rochester, New York.
HESS, A. L. and BRADSHAW, H. L. (1970). Positiveness of self-concept

and ideal self as a function of age. *Journal of Genetic Psychology,* **117**, 57.

HEWITT, S., NEWSON, J. and NEWSON, E. (1970). *The Family And The Handicapped Child.* Aldine, Chicago.

HINKLE, L. and WOLF, S. (1949). Experimental study of life situations, emotions and occurence of acidosis in a juvenile diabetic. *American Journal of the Medical Sciences,* **217**, 130.

HINKLE, L. and WOLF, S. (1952). A summary of experimental evidence relating life stress to diabetes mellitus. *Journal of Mt. Sinai Hospital,* **19**, 537.

HOLDAWAY, D. (1972). Educating the handicapped child and his parents. *Clinical Pediatrics,* **11**, 63.

HOLDEN, R. H. (1962). Changes in body image of physically handicapped children due to summer camp experience. *Merrill-Palmer Quarterly,* **8**, 19.

HOLTZMAN, W. H., THORPE, J. S., SWARTZ, J. D and HERRON, E. W. (1961). *Inkblot Perception and Personality. Holtzman Inkblot Technique.* University of Texas Press, Austin, Texas.

HONZIK, M. P., COLLART, D. S., ROBINSON, S. J. and FINLEY, K. H. (1969). Sex differences in verbal and performance IQ's of children undergoing open-heart surgery. *Science,* **164**, 445.

HOOK, E. (1973). Behavioral implications of the human XYX genotype. *Science,* **179**, 139.

HOOK, E. and KIM, D-S. (1971). Height and antisocial behavior in XY and XYY boys. *Science,* **172**, 284.

HOROWITZ, F. D. (1962). The relationship of anxiety, self-concept, and sociometric status among fourth, fifth, and sixth grade children. *Journal of Abnormal and Social Psychology,* **65**, 212.

HUNT, G. M. (1973). Implications of the treatment of myelomeningocele for the child and his family. *Lancet,* December, 1308.

HYDE, J. S. and SWARTZ, C. L. (1968). Effect of an exercise program on the perennially asthmatic child. *American Journal of Diseases of Children,* **116**, 383.

INGRAM, T. T. S. (1959). Specific developmental disorders of speech in childhood. *Brain,* **82**, 450.

INGRAM, T. T. S., JAMESON, S., ERRINGTON, J. and MITCHELL, R. G. (1964). *Living With Cerebral Palsy.* Heinemann, London.

IRETON, H. R. (1969). Psychologic problems of children with seizures. *Postgraduate Medicine,* **46**, 119.

JAN, J. E., ROBINSON, G. C. and SCOTT, E. A. (1973). A multidisciplinary approach to the problems of the multihandicapped blind child. *Canadian Medical Association Journal,* **109**, 705.

JENSEN, G. D. and KOGAN, K. L. (1962). Parental estimates of the future achievement of children with cerebral palsy. *Journal of*

Mental Deficiency Research, **6**, 56.
JERSILD, A. T. (1952). *In Search of Self.* Columbia University Teachers College, Bureau of Publications, New York.
JOHNSON, H. R. and MYHRE, S. A. (1970). Effects of testosterone on body image and behavior in Klinefelters Syndrome: a pilot study. *Developmental Medicine and Child Neurology,* **12**, 454.
JONES, M. C. (1965). Psychological correlates of somatic development. *Child Development,* **36**, 899.
KAGAN, J., HENKER, B. A., HEN-TOV, A., LEVINE, J. and LEWIS, M. (1966). Infants' differential reactions to familiar and distorted faces. *Child Development,* **37**, 518.
KAMMERER, R. C. (1940). An exploratory study of crippled children. *Psychological Record,* **4**, 47.
KANOF, A., KUTNER, B., GORDON, N. B. (1962). The impact of infantile amaurotic familial idiocy (Tay Sachs Disease) on the family. *Pediatrics,* **29**, 37.
KANTHOR, H., PLESS, B., SATTERWHITE, B. and MYERS, G. (1974). Areas of responsibility in the health care of multiply handicapped child. *Pediatrics,* **54**, 779.
KAPLAN, H. B. (1970). Self-derogation and childhood family structure: Family size, birth order, and sex distribution. *Journal of Nervous and Mental Disease,* **151**, 13.
KAPLAN, H. B. and POKORNY, A. D. (1969). Self-derogation and psychosocial adjustment. *Journal of Nervous and Mental Disease,* **149**, 421.
KAPLAN DE-NOUR, A. and CZACZKES, J. W. (1971). Professional team opinion and personal bias—a study of a chronic hemodialysis unit team. *Journal of Chronic Diseases,* **24**, 533.
KARP, M., MANOR, M. and LARON, Z. (1970). What do juvenile diabetics and their family know about diabetes? In *Habilitation and Rehabilitation of Juvenile Diabetics. Proceedings of First Beilinson Symposium on Juvenile Diabetes.* p. 83 (Z. T. Laron, ed.). Williams & Wilkins, Baltimore.
KATZ, A. H. (1963). Social adaptation in chronic illness: A study of hemophilia. *American Journal of Public Health,* **53**, 166.
KATZ, A. H. (1970). *Hemophilia—A Study in Hope and Reality.* Thomas, Springfield, Illinois.
KEARSLEY, R. B., SNIDER, M. and EATON, A. A. B. (1964). A practical quantitative method of recognizing behavioral illness in boys 9 to 14 years of age. *Journal of Pediatrics,* **65**, 256.
KEITH, R. A. and MARKIE, G. S. (1969). Parental and professional assessment of functioning in cerebral palsy. *Developmental Medicine and Child Neurology,* **11**, 735.
KELESKE, L., SOLOMONS, G. and OPITZ, E. (1967). Parental reactions

to phenylketonuria in the family. *Journal of Pediatrics*, **70**, 793.
KELLER, M. (1953). Progress in school of children in a sample of families in the eastern health district of Baltimore, Maryland. *Milbank Memorial Fund Quarterly*, **31**, 391.
KELLMER-PRINGLE, M. L. (1964). *The Emotional and Social Adjustment of Physically Handicapped Children*. Information Service of the National Foundation for Educational Research in England and Wales.
KELLMER-PRINGLE, M. L. (1974). 'Don't just research; do something.' *Observer Review*, June 9, 26.
KELLMER-PRINGLE, M. L. and FIDDES, D. O. (1970). *The Challenge of Thalidomide*. Longman, London.
KENNELL, J. H., SOROKER, E., THOMAS, P. and WASMAN, M. (1969). What parents of rheumatic fever patients don't understand about the disease and its prophylactic management. *Pediatrics*, **43**, 160.
KHAN, A. V., HERNDON, C. H. and AHMADIAN, S. Y. (1971). Social and emotional adaptations of children with transplanted kidneys and chronic hemodialysis. *American Journal of Psychiatry*, **127**, 114.
KIMBALL, C. P. (1971). Emotional and psychosocial aspects of diabetes mellitus. *Medical Clinics of North America*, **55**, 1007.
KING, S. H. (1955). Psychosocial factors associated with rheumatoid arthritis. *Journal of Chronic Diseases*, **2**, 296.
KLAPPER, Z. S and BIRCH, H. C. (1966). The relation of childhood characteristics to outcome in young adults with cerebral palsy. *Developmental Medicine and Child Neurology*, **8**, 645.
KLEIN, S. (1974). Measuring the outcome of the impact of chronic childhood illness on the family. In *Conference on the Measurement of Outcome in the Care of Children with Chronic Illness*. Fogarty International Center and the National Institutes of Child Health and Human Development, Bethesda, Maryland. (in press).
KNORR, N. J., HOOPES, J. E. and EDGERTON, M. T. (1968). Psychiatric-surgical approach to adolescent disturbance in self-image. *Plastic and Reconstructive Surgery*, **41**, 248.
KOHLBERG, I. F. and ROTHENBERG, M. B. (1970). Comprehensive care following multiple life-threatening injuries. *American Journal of Diseases of Children*, **119**, 449.
KOLODNY, R. L. and WALDFOGEL, S. (1967). Modifying tensions between the handicapped and their normal peers in group work with children. *Journal of Psychosomatic Research*, **17**, 271.
KORSCH, B. and BARNETT, H. L. (1961). The physician, the family, and the child with nephrosis. *Journal of Pediatrics*, **58**, 707.
KORSCH, B. M. and FINE, R. M. (1971). Experiences of children and their families during extended hemodialysis and kidney transplantation. *Pediatric Clinics of North America*, **18**, 625.

REFERENCES

KORSCH, B. M., FRAAD, L. and BARNETT, H. L. (1954). Pediatric discussions with parent groups. *Journal of Pediatrics*, **14**, 171.

KORSCH, B. M., GOWZI, E. K. and FRANCIS, V. (1968). Gaps in doctor-patient communication. *Pediatrics*, **42**, 855.

KORSCH, B. M., NEGRETTE, V. F., GARDNER, J. E., WEINSTOCK, C. L., MERCER, A. S., GRUSHKIN, C. M. and FINE, R. M. (1973). Kidney transplantation in children: Psychosocial follow-up study on child and family. *Journal of Pediatrics*, **83**, 399.

KOSKI, M. J. (1969). The coping processes in childhood diabetes. *Acta Paediatrica Scandinavica*, Supplement 198, p. 1.

LaFORGE, R. and SUCZEK, R. F. (1955). The interpersonal dimension personality: III — an interpersonal check list. *Journal of Personality*, **24**, 94.

LaHOOD, B. J. (1970). Parental attitudes and their influence on the medical management of diabetic adolescents. *Clinical Pediatrics*, **9**, 468.

LAMBERT, C. N., HAMILTON, R. C. and PELLICORE, R. J. (1969). The juvenile amputee program: Its social and economic value. *Journal of Bone and Joint Surgery*, **51-A**, 1135.

LANDTMAN, B., VALANNE, E. H. and AUKEE, M. (1968). Emotional complications of heart disease. A study of 256 children with real and 'imaginary' heart disease. *Annales Paediatriae Finniae*, **14**, 71.

LANDTMAN, B., VALANNE, E. H., PENTTI, R. and AUKEE, M. (1960). Psychosomatic behaviour of children with congenital heart disease. *Annales Paediatric Finniae*, Supplement 15, 6.

LAPOUSE, R. and MONK, M. A. (1958). An epidemiological study of behavioral characteristics in children. *American Journal of Public Health*, **48**, 1134.

LANCET, (1966). Cardiac neurosis in children (Annotation). *Lancet*, **ii**, 430.

LARON, Z. T. (1970). *Habilitation and Rehabilitation of Juvenile Diabetes. Proceedings of the First Beilinson Symposium on Juvenile Diabetes.* Williams & Wilkins, Baltimore.

LAURENCE, K. M. and TEW, B. J. (1969). Follow-up of 65 survivors from the 425 cases of spina bifida born in South Wales between 1956 and 1962. In *Research into Hydrocephalus and Spina Bifida, Developmental Medicine and Child Neurology*, Supplement 13, 1.

LAWLER, R. H., NAKIELNY, W. and WRIGHT, N. Y. (1966). Psychological implications of cystic fibrosis. *Canadian Medical Association Journal*, **94**, 1043.

LAZARUS, R. S. (1966). *Psychological Stress and the Coping Process.* McGraw-Hill, New York.

LEVINE, E. S. (1951). Psychoeducational study of children born deaf

following maternal rubella in pregnancy. *American Journal of Diseases of Children,* **81,** 627.
LEVINE, E. S. (1971). Mental assessment of the deaf child. *Volta Review,* February, 80.
LEVY, N. (1958). A short form of the children's manifest anxiety scale. *Child Development,* **29,** 153.
LEWIN, K. (1936). *Principles of Topological Psychology.* McGraw-Hill, New York.
LEWIS, C. (1971). Does comprehensive care make a difference: what is the evidence? *American Journal of Diseases of Children,* **122,** 469.
LINDE, L. M., ROSOF, B., DUNN, O. J. and RABB, E. (1966). Attitudinal factors in congenital heart disease. *Pediatrics,* **38,** 92.
LINDE, L. M., ROSOF, B., and DUNN, O. J. (1970). Longitudinal studies of intellectual and behavioral development in children with congenital heart disease. *Acta Paediatrica Scandinavica,* **59,** 169.
LINDER, R. (1970). Mothers of disabled children—the value of weekly group meetings.*Developmental Medicine and Child Neurology,* **12,** 202.
LIPOWSKI, Z. J. (1970). Physical illness, the individual and the coping process. *Psychiatry in Medicine,* **1,** 91.
LIPSETT, L. P. (1958). A self-concept scale for children and its relationship to the children's form of the manifest anxiety scale. *Child Development,* **29,** 463.
LONG, B. H., HENDERSON, E. H. and ZILLER, R. C. (1967). Developmental changes in the self-concept during middle childhood. *Merrill-Palmer Quarterly,* **13,** 201.
LOVE, H. D. (1970). *Parental Attitudes Toward Exceptional Children.* Thomas, Springfield, Illinois.
LOWIT, I. (1973). Social and psychological consequences of chronic illness in children. *Developmental Medicine and Child Neurology,* **15,** 75.
McANARNEY, E., PLESS, I. B., SATTERWHITE, B. and FRIEDMAN, S. (1974). Psychological problems of children with chronic juvenile arthritis. *Pediatrics,* **53,** 523.
McCLURE, W. J. (1966). Current problems and trends in the education of the deaf. *Deaf American,* **18,** 8.
McCOLLUM, A. T. and GIBSON, L. E. (1970). Family adaptation to the child with cystic fibrosis. *Journal of Pediatrics,* **77,** 571.
McCRAE, W. M., CULL, A. M. BURTON, L. and DODGE, J. (1973). Cystic fibrosis: parents' response to the genetic basis of the disease. *Lancet,* **3,** 141.
McCRAW, R. M. and TRAVIS, L. B. (1973). Psychological effects of a special summer camp on juvenile diabetics. *Diabetes,* **22,** 275.

REFERENCES

McDANIEL, J. W. (1969). *Physical Disability and Human Behaviour.* Pergamon Press, London.

McFIE, J. and ROBERTSON, J. (1973). Psychological test results of children with thalidomide deformities. *Developmental Medicine and Child Neurology,* **15**, 719.

McLEAN, J. A., SCHRAGER, J., STOEFFLER, V. R. and ARBOR, A. (1968). Severe asthma in children. *Michigan Medicine,* **67**, 1219.

McMICHAEL, J.(1971). *Handicap: A Study of Physically Handicapped Children And Their Families.* Staples Press, London.

MACGREGOR, F. (1951). Some psycho-social problems associated with facial deformities. *American Sociological Review,* **16**, 629.

MACGREGOR, F. (1963). Facial disfigurement and problems of employment: Some social and cultural considerations. In *Facial Disfigurement: A Rehabilitation Problem* (B. O. Rogers, ed.). US Department of Health, Education, and Welfare, Washington.

MACGREGOR, F. C., ABEL, T. M., BRYT, A., LAUER, E. and WEISSMAN, S. (1953). *Facial Deformities and Plastic Surgery.* Thomas, Springfield, Illinois.

MACHOVER, K. (1949). *Personality Projection In The Drawing Of The Human Figure.* Thomas, Springfield, Illinois.

MACHOVER, K. (1951). Drawings of the human figure: A method of personality investigation. In *An Introduction to Projective Techniques,* (Anderson, H. A. and Anderson, G. L. eds.). Prentice Hall, New York.

MADDISON, D. and RAPHAEL, B. (1971). Social and psychological consequences of chronic disease in childhood. *Medical Journal of Australia,* **2**, 1265.

MAHRER, A. (1969). Childhood determinants of adult functioning: Strategies in the clinical research use of the personal-psychological history. *Psychological Record,* **19**, 39.

MARGE, D. K. (1966). The social status of speech-handicapped children. *Journal of Speech and Hearing Research,* **9**, 166.

MARTIN, H. L. (1969). The significance of discussion with patients about their diagnosis and its implication. *British Journal of Medical Psychology,* **40**, 233.

MASON, J. (1954). Suicide in adolescents. *Psychoanalytic Review,* **41**, 48.

MATTSSON, A. (1972). Long-term physical illness in childhood: A challenge to psychosocial adaptation. *Pediatrics,* **50**, 801.

MATTSSON, A. and AGLE, D. (1972). Group therapy with the parents of hemophiliacs: Therapeutic process and observations of parental adaptation to chronic illness in children. *Journal of the American Academy of Child Psychiatry,* **11**, 558.

MATTSSON, A. and GROSS, S. (1966). Adaptational and defensive behavior in young hemophiliacs and their parents. *American Journal of Psychiatry,* **122,** 1349.

MATTSSON, A., GROSS, S. and HALL, T. W. (1971). Psychoendocrine study of adaptation in young hemophiliacs. *Psychosomatic Medicine,* **XXXIII,** 215.

MAXWELL, G. M. and GANE, S. (1962). The impact of congenital heart disease upon the family. *American Heart Journal,* **64,** 449.

MEADOW, K. P. (1969). Parental response to the medical ambiguities of congenital deafness. *Journal of Health and Social Behavior,* **19,** 299.

MECHANIC, D. (1968). *Medical Sociology—A Selective View.* Free Press, New York.

MERRILL, R. E. (1971). Prognosis for children with multiple handicaps. *American Journal of Diseases of Children,* **121,** 207.

MEYEROWITZ, J. H. and KAPLAN, H. B. (1967). Familial responses to stress: the care of cystic fibrosis. *Social Science and Medicine,* **1,** 249.

MILMAN, D. H. (1952). Group therapy with parents: An approach to the rehabilitation of physically disabled children. *Journal of Pediatrics,* **41,** 113.

MINDE, K., HACKETT, J. D., KILLOU, D. and SILVER, S. (1972). How they grow up: 41 physically handicapped children and their families. *American Journal of Psychiatry,* **128,** 12.

MINDE, K. and MALER, L. (1968). Psychiatric counseling on a pediatric medical ward: a controlled evaluation. *Journal of Pediatrics,* **72,** 452.

MITCHELL, R. G. (1971). The prevention of cerebral palsy. *Developmental Medicine and Child Neurology,* **13,** 137.

MOLDOFSKY, H. and ROTHMAN, A. I. (1970). Personality, disease parameters, and medication in rheumatoid arthritis. *Arthritis and Rheumatism,* **13,** 388.

MONBECK, M. E. (1973). *The Meaning of Blindness—Attitudes Toward Blindness and Blind People.* Indiana University Press, Bloomington, Indiana.

MONEY, J. and POLLITT, E. (1966). Studies in the psychology of dwarfism II. Personality maturation and response to growth hormone treatment in hypopitutitary dwarfs. *Journal of Pediatrics,* **68,** 381.

MOOS, R. H. and SOLOMON, G. F. (1964). Personality correlates of the degree of functional incapacity of patients with physical disease. *Journal of Chronic Diseases,* **18,** 1019.

MORSE, J. (1965). Making hospitalization a growth experience for arthritic children. *Social Casework,* **46,** 550.

MORSE, J. (1968). Involving fathers in the treatment of patients with

juvenile rheumatoid arthritis. *Social Casework,* **49,** 281.
MORSE, J. (1972). Aspiration and achievement — A study of one hundred patients with juvenile rheumatoid arthritis. *Rehabilitation Literature,* **33,** 290.
MORSE, J. (1974). Family involvement in pediatric dialysis and transplantation. *Social Casework,* **55,** 216.
MORSE, J., SEGLIN, J., BURNSIDE, M. and GLODE, G. (1966). Teamwork in a center for juvenile rheumatoid arthritis. *Rehabilitation Literature,* **27,** 258.
MURAWSKI, B. J., CHAZAN, B. I., BALODIMOS, M. C. and RYAN, J. R. (1970). Personality patterns in patients with diabetes mellitus of long duration. *Diabetes,* **19,** 259.
MUSSEN, P. and NEWMAN, D. K. (1958). Handicap, motivation, and adjustment in physically disabled children. *Exceptional Children,* **24,** 255.
MUTHARD, J. E. (1965). MMPI findings for cerebral palsied college students. *Journal of Consulting Psychology,* **29,** 599.
MYERS, B. A., FRIEDMAN, S. B. and WEINER, I. B. (1970). Coping with a chronic disability. *American Journal of Diseases of Children,* **120,** 175.
NEUHAUS, E. C. (1958). A personality study of asthmatic and cardiac children. *Psychosomatic Medicine,* **XX,** 181.
NEUHAUS, M. (1969). Parental attitudes and the emotional adjustment of deaf children. *Exceptional Children,* **35,** 721.
NEWSON, J. and NEWSON, E. (1969). *Four Years Old in an Urban Community.* Allen & Unwin, London.
NIELSON, H. H. (1971). Psychological appraisal of children with cerebral palsy: A survey of 128 re-assessed cases. *Developmental Medicine and Child Neurology,* **13,** 707.
NIELSON, J. and TSUBOI, T. (1970). Correlation between stature, character disorder and criminality. *British Journal of Psychiatry,* **116,** 145.
NOLAND, R. L. (1971). *Counseling Parents of the Ill and the Handicapped.* Thomas, Springfield, Illinois.
NOWLIS, V. and NOWLIS, H. (1956). The description and analysis of mood. *Annals of the New York Academy of Sciences,* **65,** 345.
OFFER, D. and SABSHIN, M. (1966). *Normality: Theoretical and Clinical Concepts of Mental Health.* Basic Books, New York.
OLCH, D. (1971a). Effects of hemophilia upon intellectual growth and academic achievement. *Journal of Genetic Psychology,* **119,** 63.
OLCH, D. (1971b). Personality characteristics of hemophiliacs. *Journal of Personality Assessment,* **35,** 72.
O'REILLY, D. E. (1971). The future of the cerebral palsied child. *Developmental Medicine and Child Neurology,* **13,** 635.

OSGOOD, C. E., SUCI, G. J. and TANNENBAUM, P. H. (1957). *The Measurement of Meaning.* University of Illinois Press, Chicago.

OUNSTED, C., LINDSAY, J. and NORMAN, R. (1966). Biological factors in temporal lobe epilepsy. *Clinics in Developmental Medicine,* **22**, 135.

PARMALEE, A. H. and WOLFF, P. (1966). Developmental studies of blind children. *New Outlook for the Blind,* **46**, 177.

PATTERSON, P. R., DENNING, C. R. and KUTSCHER, A. H. (1973). *Psychosocial Aspects of Cystic Fibrosis—A Model for Chronic Lung Disease.* Columbia University Press, New York.

PEABODY, F. W. (1927). Care of patient. *Journal of the American Medical Association,* **88**, 877.

PERKINS, H. V. (1958). Teachers' and peers' perceptions of children's self-concepts. *Child Development,* **29**, 203.

PERRIN, R. P., RUSCH, E. L., PRAY, J. L., WRIGHT, G. F. and BARTLETT, G. S. (1972). Evaluation of a ten year experience in a comprehensive care program for handicapped children. *Pediatrics,* **50**, 793.

PESHKIN, M. M. (1930). Asthma in children—The role of environment in the treatments of a selected group of cases: A plea for a 'home' as a restorative measure. *American Journal of Diseases of Children,* **38**, 774.

PETERSON, K. H. and McELHENNEY, T. R. (1965). Effects of a physical fitness program upon asthmatic boys. *Pediatrics,* **35**, 295.

PIERS, E. V. (1969). *Manual for the Piers-Harris Children's Self Concept Scale (The Way I Feel About Myself).* Counselor Recordings and Tests, Nashville, Tenn.

PIERS, E. V. and HARRIS, D. B. (1964). Age and other correlates of self-concept in children. *Journal of Educational Psychology,* **55**, 91.

PILLING, D. (1973). *The Child With A Chronic Medical Problem—Cardiac Disorders, Diabetes, Haemophilia.* National Children's Bureau Report, NFER Publishing Co. Ltd., Slough.

PINKERTON, P. (1969). Managing the psychological aspects of cystic fibrosis. *Arizona Medicine,* **26**, 348.

PINKERTON, P. (1970a). Parental acceptance of the handicapped child. *Developmental Medicine and Child Neurology,* **12**, 207.

PINKERTON, P. (1970b). The influence of sociopathology in childhood asthma. *Psychotherapy and Psychosomatics,* **18**, 231.

PINKERTON, P. and WEAVER, C. M. (1970). Childhood asthma. In *Modern Trends in Psychosomatic Medicine, 2nd Series.* Butterworth, London.

PINKERTON, P., WEAVER, C. M. and HENRY, K. (1971). Reappraisal of parentectory in childhood asthma. *Medical Officer,* **125**, 63.

PINKERTON, P. (1971a). Depression vs. denial in childhood asthma: Equipotent fatal hazards. In *Depressive States in Childhood and*

Adolescents, p. 187, (Annell, A., ed.). Almqvist and Wiksell, Stockholm.

PINKERTON, P. (1971b). Childhood asthma. *British Journal of Hospital Medicine*, 6, 331.

PINKERTON, P. (1971c). Psychosomatic inter-relationships in the management of childhood asthma. *Psychotherapy and Psychosomatics*, 19, 257.

PINKERTON, P. (1973). Paediatrics and child psychiatry. *Archives of Disease in Childhood*, 48, 970.

PINKERTON, P. (1974a). Inpatient treatment of children with psychosomatic disorder. In *The Residential Psychiatric Treatment of Children*, (Barker, P., ed.). Crosby Lockwood Staples, London.

PINKERTON, P. (1974b). What is a psychosomatic disorder? *Update*, 8, 475.

PINKERTON, P. (1974c). Psychological problems of children with chronic illness. In *The Care of Children with Chronic Illness. Proceedings of 67th Conference on Pediatric Research*. Ross Laboratories, Columbus, Ohio (in press).

PLESS, I. B. (1966). Chronic disease in childhood — A new challenge. *St. Mary's Hospital Gazette*, 211.

PLESS, I. B. (1969). Why special education for physically handicapped pupils? *Social and Economic Administration*, 3, 253.

PLESS, I. B., CHERRY, N. M., DOUGLAS, J. W. B. and WADSWORTH, M. E. J. (1975). Psychological and social aspects of long-term illness in childhood: Results from a longitudinal national survey. Unpublished manuscript.

PLESS, I. B. and DOUGLAS, J. W. B. (1971). Chronic illness in childhood: I. Epidemiological and clinical characteristics. *Pediatrics*, 47, 405.

PLESS, I. B., RACKHAM, K. and KELLOCK, T. D. (1967). Patterns in the admission of handicapped pupils to residential establishments. *Medical Officer*, 118, 135.

PLESS. I. B. and ROGHMANN, K. J. (1971). Chronic illness and its consequences: Observations based on three epidemiological surveys. *Journal of Pediatrics*, 79, 351.

PLESS, I. B., ROGHMANN, K. J. and HAGGERTY, R. J. (1972). Chronic illness, family functioning, and psychological adjustment: A model for the allocation of preventive mental health services. *International Journal of Epidemiology*, 1, 271.

PLESS, I. B. and SATTERWHITE, B. (1971). Health education literature for parents of handicapped children. *American Journal of Diseases of Children*, 122, 206.

PLESS, I. B. and SATTERWHITE, B. (1972). Chronic illness in child-

hood: Selection, activities, and evaluation of non-professional family counselors. *Clinical Pediatrics,* 11, 403.
PLESS, I. B. and SATTERWHITE, B. (1973). A measure of family functioning and its application. *Social Science and Medicine,* 7, 613.
PLESS, I. B. and SATTERWHITE, B. (1975). Chronic illness, In *Child Health and the Community,* (Haggerty, R. J., Roghmann, K. J. and Pless, I. B., eds.). Wiley, New York.
POLLITT, E. and MONEY, J. (1964). Studies in the psychology of dwarfism. I. Intelligence quotient and school achievement. *Journal of Pediatrics,* 64, 415.
POLLOCK, G. A. and STARK, G. (1969). Long-term results in the management of 67 children with cerebral palsy. *Developmental Medicine and Child Neurology,* 11, 17.
PORTER, R. B. and ATTELL, R. S. (1959). *Children's Personality Questionnaire.* USA Institute of Personality Testing, Washington.
POZNANSKI, E. O. (1973). Emotional issues in raising handicapped children. *Rehabilitation Literature,* 34, 322.
PURCELL, K. (1963). Distinctions between subgroups of asthmatic children. Children's perceptions of events associated with asthma. *Pediatrics,* 32, 486.
PURCELL, K., BRADY, K., CHAI, H., MUSER, J., MOLK, L., GORDON, N and MEANS, J. (1969). The effect on asthma in children of experimental separation from the family. *Psychosomatic Medicine,* **XXXI**, 144.
PURCELL, K and METZ, J. P. (1962). Distinctions between subgroups of asthmatic children: Some parent attitude variables selected to age of onset of asthma. *Journal of Psychosomatic Research,* 6, 251.
PURCELL, K., MUSER, L., MIKLICH, D and DIETIKER, K. E. (1969). A comparison of psychologic findings in variously defined asthmatic subgroups. *Journal of Psychosomatic Research,* 13, 67.
QUAY, H. D. and PETERSON, D. R. (1967). *Manual for the Behavior Problem Checklist.* University of Illinois Press, Champaign, Illinois.
RAINER, J. D., ALTSCHULER, K. Z. and KALLMAN, F. J. (1963). *Family and Mental Health Problems on a Deaf Population.* Columbia University Press, New York.
RAINER, J. D. and ALTSCHULER, K. Z. (1966). *Comprehensive Mental Health Services for the Deaf.* Columbia University Press, New York.
RAINER, J. D. and ALTSCHULER, K. Z. (1970). *Expanded Mental Health Care for the Deaf: Rehabilitation and Prevention.* New York State Psychiatric Institute, New York.
REED, A. E. and CANTONI, L. J. (1966). Employment status of handicapped college graduates. *New Outlook for the Blind,* 60,

266.
REITE, M., DAVIS, K., SOLOMONS, C. and OTT, J. (1972). Osteogenesis imperfecta: psychological function. *American Journal of Psychiatry*, **128**, 90.
REIVICH, R. S. and ROTHROCK, I. A. (1972). Behavior problems of deaf children and adolescents: A factory-analytic study. *Journal of Speech and Hearing Research*, **15**, 93.
REYNELL, J. K. (1965). Post-operative disturbances observed in children with cerebral palsy. *Developmental Medicine and Child Neurology*, **7**, 360.
RICHARDS, I. D. G. and McINTOSH, H. T. (1973). Spina bifida survivors and their parents: A study of problems and services. *Developmental Medicine and Child Neurology*, **15**, 293.
RICHARDS, M. (1969). The role of social worker in counselling and support. *Developmental Medicine and Child Neurology*, **11**, 786.
RICHARDSON, D. and FRIEDMAN, S. (1974). Psychosocial problems of the adolescent patient with epilepsy. *Clinical Pediatrics*, **13**, 121.
RICHARDSON, S. (1963). Some social psychological consequences of handicapping. *Pediatrics*, **32**, 291.
RICHARDSON, S. (1968). The effect of physical disability on the socialization of a child. In *A Handbook in Socialization Theory*. p. 1047 (Goslin, D. A. and Glass, D. C. eds.). Rand McNally, New York.
RICHARDSON, S. (1972). People with cerebral palsy talk for themselves. *Developmental Medicine and Child Neurology*, **14**, 524.
RICHARDSON, S., HASTORF, A. H. and DORNBUSCH, S. M. (1964). Effects of physical disability on a child's description of himself. *Child Development*, **35**, 93.
RICHARDSON, S., HASTORF, A. H., GOODMAN, N. and DORNBUSCH, S. M. (1961). Cultural uniformity in reactions to physical disabilities. *American Sociological Review*, **26**, 241.
RIE, H. E., BOVERMAN, H., OZOA, N. and GROSSMAN, B. J. (1964). Tutoring and ventilation. *Clinical Pediatrics*, **3**, 581.
RILEY, C. M. (1964). Thoughts about kidney transplantation in children. *Journal of Pediatrics*, **65**, 797.
ROBACK, H. B. (1968). Human figure drawings: Their utility in the clinical psychologist's armamentation for personality assessment. *Psychological Bulletin*, **70**, 1.
ROBINSON, H., KIRK, R. F. and FRYE, R. L. (1971). A psychological study of rheumatoid arthritis and selected controls. *Journal of Chronic Diseases*, **23**, 791.
RODDA, M. (1970). *The Hearing-impaired School Leaver*. University of London Press, London.
ROGERS, C. R. (1951). *Client-Centred Therapy*. Houghton-Mifflin,

Boston.
ROGERS, C. R. and DYMOND, R. F. (1954). *Psychotherapy and Personality Change.* University of Chicago Press, Chicago.
ROSEN, H. and LIDZ, T. (1949). Emotional factors in the precipitation in the recurrent diabetic acidosis. *Psychosomatic Medicine,* **11**, 211.
ROSENBERG, M. (1965). *Society and the Adolescent Self-Image.* Princeton University Press, Princeton, New Jersey.
ROSENZWEIG, S. (1948). Picture-frustration test. In *Exploration of Personality,* (Murrary, H. A., ed.). Oxford University Press, New York.
ROSKIES, E. (1972). *Abnormality and Normality: The Mothering of Thalidomide Children.* Cornell University Press, Ithaca, New York.
ROTTER, J. B. (1950). *Incomplete Sentence Blank.* Psychological Corp, New York.
RUBIN, R. A., ROSENBLATT, C. and BALOW, B. (1973). Psychological and educational sequelae of prematurity. *Pediatrics,* **52**, 352.
RUSSAK, S. and FRIEDMAN, D. B. (1970). Family interviewing and pediatric training. *Clinical Pediatrics,* **9**, 594.
RUTTER, M. and GRAHAM, P. (1970). Psychiatric aspects of intellectual and educational retardation. In *Education, Health and Behaviour,* p. 102, (Rutter, M., Tizard, J. and Whitmore, K. eds.). Longman, London.
RUTTER, M., GRAHAM, P. and YULE, W. (1970). *A Neuropsychiatric Study in Childhood.* Spastics International Medical Publications, Heinemann Medical Books, London.
RUTTER, M., TIZARD, J. and WHITMORE, K., eds. (1970). *Education, Health and Behaviour.* Longman, London.
SACKS, L., FERNSTEIN, A. R. and TARANTA, A. (1962). A controlled psychological study of Sydenham's chorea. *Journal of Pediatrics,* **61**, 714.
SAFFLIOS-ROTHSCHILD, C. (1970). *The Sociology and Social Psychology of Disability.* Random House, New York.
SALK, L., HILGARTNER, N. and GRANICH, B. (1972). The psychosocial impact of hemophilia on the patient and his family. *Social Science and Medicine,* **6**, 491.
SARASON, S. B., DAVIDSON, K. S., LIGHTHALL, F. F. and WAITE, R. R. (1958). A test anxiety scale for children. *Child Development,* **29**, 105.
SCHEIN, J. D. and BUSHNAQ, S. (1962). Higher education for the deaf in the United States—retrospective investigation. *American Annals of the Deaf,* **107**, 416.
SCHERZER, A. L. and GARDNER, G. G. (1971). Studies of the school age

child with meningomyelocele: I. Physical and intellectual development. *Pediatrics*, **47**, 424.
SCHILDER, P. (1950). *The Image and Appearance of the Human Body*. International University Press, New York.
SCHLESINGER, H. S. and MEADOW, K. P. (1972). *Sound and Sigh—Childhood Deafness and Mental Health*. University of California Press, Berkeley, California.
SCHOGGEN, P. (1974). An ecological study of children with physical disability in school and at home. In *Systematic Observations in School Settings*, (Weinberg, R., ed.). University of Minnesota Press, Minneapolis (in press).
SCHOENFELD, W. A. (1964). Body-image disturbances in adolescents with inappropriate sexual development. *American Journal of Orthopsychiatry*, **XXXIV**, 493.
SCHWAB, J. J. and HARMELING, J. D. M. A. (1968). Body image and medical illness. *Psychosomatic Medicine*, **XXX**, 51.
SEARS, P. S. (1971). Self concept inventory. In *Tests and Measurements in Child Development—A Handbook*, (Johnson, O. G. and Bommarito, J. W., eds.). Josey-Bass, San Francisco.
SECORD, P. F. and JOURARD, S. M. (1953). The appraisal of body-cathexis: Body-cathexis and self. *Journal of Consulting and Clinical Psychology*, **17**, 343.
SEIDENFELD, M. A. (1948). The psychological sequelae of poliomyelitis in children. *Nervous Child*, **7**, 14.
SHERE, M. O. (1956). Socio-emotional factors in the family of twins with cerebral palsy. *Exceptional Children*, **22**, 196.
SHERE, E. and KASTENBAUM, K. (1966). Mother-child interaction in cerebral palsy: Environmental and psychosocial obstacles to cognitive development. *Genetic Psychology Monographs*, **73**, 255.
SHRUT, A. (1964). Suicidal adolescents and children. *Journal of the American Medical Association*, **188**, 1103.
SIBINGA, M. S. and FRIEDMAN, C. J. (1971). Complexities of parental understanding of phenylketonuria. *Pediatrics*, **48**, 216.
SIEGELMAN, E., BLOCK, J., BLOCK, J. and VON DER LIPPE, A. (1970). Antecedents of optimal psychological adjustment. *Journal of Consulting and Clinical Psychology*, **35**, 283.
SILLER, J. (1960). Psychological concomitants of amputation in children. *Child Development*, **31**, 109.
SIMMONS, R. G., ROSENBERG, F. and ROSENBERG, M. (1973). Disturbance in the self-image at adolescence. *American Sociological Review*, **38**, 553.
SIMPSON, M. (1964). Survey of children born in 1947 who were in schools for the deaf in 1962-3. In *The Health of the School Child, Report of the Chief Medical Officer 1962 & 1963*. HMSO, London.

SMARS, G. and BERFENSTRAM, A. (1961). *Osteogenesis Imperfecta in Sweden*. Scandinavian University Books, Stockholm.
SMITH, L. (1958). The concurrent validity of six personality and adjustment tests for children. *Psychological Monographs; General and Applied*, **72**, 1.
SMITH, R. M. and McWILLIAMS, B. J. (1966). Creative thinking abilities of cleft palate children. *Cleft Palate Journal*, **3**, 275.
SMITH, R. M. and McWILLIAMS, B. J. (1968). Psycholinguistic abilities of children with clefts. *Cleft Palate Journal*, **5**, 238.
SMITHELLS, R. W. (1969). The management of congenital abnormality. *British Journal of Hospital Medicine*, **2**, 432.
SOLOW, C., SILDERFARB, P. M. and SWIFE, K. (1974). Psychosocial effects of intestinal bypass surgery for severe obesity. *New England Journal of Medicine*, **290**, 300.
SOMERS, V. S. (1944). *The Influence of Parental Attitudes and Social Environment in the Personality Development of the Adolescent Blind*. American Foundation For The Blind, New York.
SPENCER, R. F. (1968). Incidence of social and psychiatric problems in a group of hemophiliac patients. *North Carolina Medical Journal*, **29**, 332.
SPENCER, R. F. and BEHAR, L. (1969). Adaptation in hemophiliac adolescents. *Psychosomatics*, **10**, 304.
SPRIESTERSBACH, D. C. (1973). *Psychological Aspects of the 'Cleft Palate Problem'*. University of Iowa Press, Iowa City, Iowa.
STARFIELD, B. and BORKOWF, S. (1969). Physician's recognition of complaints made by parents about their children's health. *Pediatrics*, **43**, 168.
STEARNS, S. (1959). Self-destructive behavior in young patients with diabetes mellitus. *Diabetes*, **8**, 379.
STEHBENS, J. A. and MACQUEEN, J. C. (1973). The psychological adjustment of rheumatic fever patients with and without chorea. *Clinical Pediatrics*. **11**, 638.
STEIN, S. P. and CHARLES, E. (1971). Emotional factors in juvenile diabetes mellitus: A study of early life experience of adolescent diabetics. *American Journal of Psychiatry*, **128**, 6.
STEPHEN, E. (1963). Intelligence levels and educational status of children with meningomyelocele. *Developmental Medicine and Child Neurology*, **5**, 572.
STEPHENSON, W. (1953). *The Study of Behavior*. University of Chicago Press, Chicago.
STERKY, G. (1963). Family background and state of mental health in a group of diabetic schoolchildren. *Acta Paediatrica*, **52**, 377.
STONE, J. B. (1958). *Manual of S. O. Rorschach Test*. California Test Bureau, Los Angeles, Calif.

REFERENCES

STONE, N. D. and PARNICKEY, J. J. (1966). Factors in child placement: Parental response to congenital defect. *Social Work*, **11**, 35.

STOTT, A. (1966). *The Social Adjustment of Children*, 3rd ed. University of London Press, London.

SULLIVAN, H. S. (1954). *The Psychiatric Interview.* Norton, New York.

SULTZ, H., SCHLESINGER, E. R., MOSHER, W. E. and FELDMAN, J. G. (1972). *Long-Term Childhood Illness,* p. 116. University of Pittsburgh Press, Pittsburgh, Penna.

SUSSMAN, M. B. (1966). Sociological theory and deafness: Problems and prospects. *ASHA: Journal of American Speech and Hearing Association*, **8**, 303.

SWIFT, C., SEIDMAN, F. and STEIN, H. (1967). Adjustment problems in juvenile diabetes. *Psychosomatic Medicine*, **29**, 555.

SYMONDS, P. M. (1964). *Symonds Picture Story Test.* Teachers College, Columbia University, New York.

TAFT, L. T. (1973). The care and management of the child with muscular dystrophy. *Developmental Medicine and Child Neurology*, **15**, 510.

TARTER, R. E. (1972). Intellectual and adaptive functioning in epilepsy — A review of 50 years of work. *Diseases of the Nervous System*, **33**, 763.

TAULBEE, E. S. and STENMARK, D. (1968). The Blacky Pictures Test: A Comprehensive annotated and indexed bibliography. *Journal of Projective Techniques and Personality Assessment*, **32**, 105.

TAYLOR, C. and COMBS, A. W. (1952). Self acceptance and adjustment. *Journal of Consulting Psychology*, **16**, 89.

TAYLOR, J. A. (1953). A personality scale of manifest anxiety. *Journal of Abnormal and Social Psychology*, **48**, 285.

TEW, B. J. and LAURENCE, K. M. (1973). Mothers, brothers and sisters of patients with spina bifida. *Developmental Medicine and Child Neurology*, **15**, Supplement 29, 69.

THELANDER, H. E. (1968). Prognosis of children with 'cerebral palsy'. Reflections on stock-taking. *Clinical Pediatrics*, **7**, 294.

THOMAS, L. A., MILMAN, D. H. and RODRIQUEZ-TORRES, R. (1970). Anxiety in children with rheumatic fever: Relation to route of prophylaxis. *Journal of the American Medical Association*, **212**, 2080.

THORPE, L. P., CLARK, W. W. and TIEGS, E. W. (1953). *California Test of Personality.* California Test Bureau, McGraw-Hill, San Francisco.

TIETZ, W and VIDMAR, J. T. (1972). The impact of coping styles on the control of juvenile diabetes. *Psychiatry in Medicine*, **3**, 67.

TIZARD, J. and GRAD, J. C. (1961). *The Mentally Handicapped And Their Families—A Social Survey.* Oxford University Press, London.

TRAPP, E. P. and HIMMELSTEIN, P. (1962). *Readings on the Exceptional Child.* Methuen, London.

TREUTING, F. (1962). The role of emotional factors in the etiology and course of diabetes mellitus: A review of the recent literature. *American Journal of the Medical Sciences,* **244**, 93.

TROPAUER, A., FRANZ, M. N. and DILGARD, V. W. (1970). Psychological aspects of the care of children with cystic fibrosis. *American Journal of Diseases of Children,* **119**, 424.

TRAUX, C. B. and CARKHAUF, R. R. (1967). *Toward Effective Counseling and Psychotherapy: Training and Practice.* Aldine, Chicago.

TURK, J. (1964). Impact of cystic fibrosis in family functioning. *Pediatrics,* **34**, 67.

UNDERBERG, R. P., VERILLO, R. T., BENHAM, F. C. and COWEN, E. L. (1961). Factors relating to adjustment to visual disability in adolescence. *New Outlook for the Blind,* **55**, 254.

VEGELY, A. B. and ELLIOTT, L. L. (1968). Applicability of a standardized personality test to a hearing-impaired population. *American Annals of the Deaf,* **113**, 858.

VERNON, M. (1967a). Characteristics associated with post-rubella deaf children; psychological, educational and physical. *Volta Review,* **69**, 176.

VERNON, M. (1967b). Prematurity and deafness: The magnitude and nature of the problem among deaf children. *Exceptional Children,* **33**, 289.

VERNON, M. (1969a). *Multiply Handicapped Deaf Children: Medical Education and Psychological Considerations.* Council for Exceptional Children Research Monograph, Washington, D.C.

VERNON, M. (1969b). Sociological and psychological factors associated with hearing loss. *Journal of Speech and Hearing Research,* **12**, 541.

VERNON, M. (1970). Potential, achievement, and rehabilitation in the deaf population. *Rehabilitation Literature,* **31**, 258.

VIGLIANO, A., HART, L. W. and SINGER, F. (1964). Psychiatric sequelae of old burns in children and their parents. *American Journal of Orthopsychiatry,* **XXXIV**, 753.

VIGNOS, P. J., Jr., THOMPSON, H. M., KATZ, W., MOSKOWITZ, R. W., FINK, W. and SVEC, K. H. (1972). Comprehensive care and psychosocial factors in rehabilitation in chronic rheumatoid arthritis: A controlled study. *Journal of Chronic Diseases,* **25**, 457.

VOELLER, K. K. S. and ROTHENBERG, M. B. (1973). Psychosocial aspects of the management of seizures in children, *Pediatrics,* **51**, 1072.

WALKER, J. H., THOMAS, M. and RUSSELL, I. T. (1971). Spina bifida — and the parents. *Developmental Medicine and Child Neurology,* **13**, 462.

WARD, D. (1971). Rheumatoid arthritis and personality: A controlled study. *British Medical Journal,* **2**, 297.

WEIL, W. B., Jr. and SUSSMAN, M. B. (1961). Behavior, diet and glucosuria of diabetic children in a summer camp. *Pediatrics,* **27**, 118.

WEINBERG, S. (1970). Suicidal intent in adolescence: A hypothesis about the role of physical illness. *Journal of Pediatrics,* **77**, 579.

WEINER, F. (1973). *Help For The Handicapped Child.* McGraw-Hill, New York.

WEINER, I. B. and GOLDBERG, R. W. (1974). Psychological testing of children. *Pediatric Clinics of North America,* **21**, 175.

WERDELIN, I. (1969). A study of the relationship between teacher ratings, peer ratings and self-ratings of behaviour in school. *Scandinavian Journal of Educational Research,* **13**, 147.

WERTHEIMER, N. M. (1963). A psychiatric follow-up of children with rheumatic fever and other chronic diseases. *Journal of Chronic Diseases,* **16**, 223.

WILLIAMS, C. (1968). Behavior disorders in handicapped children. *Developmental Medicine and Child Neurology,* **10**, 736.

WILLIAMS, C. (1970). Some psychiatric observations on a group of maladjusted deaf children. *Journal of Child Psychology and Psychiatry and Allied Disciplines,* **11**, 1.

WILLIAMS, C. (1973). Societal implications. In *Proceedings of the 65th Ross Conference on Pediatric Research,* (Stahlmann, M., ed.). Ross Laboratories, Columbus, Ohio.

WITTENBORN, J. R. (1961). Contributions and current status of Q methodology. *Psychological Bulletin,* **58**, 132.

WOLFF, B. B. (1971). Current psychosocial concepts in rheumatoid arthritis. *Bulletin on Rheumatic Diseases,* **22**, 656.

WOLFF, H. H. (1971). The therapeutic and developmental functions of psychotherapy. *British Journal of Medical Psychology,* **44**, 117.

WOLFF, P. (1966). Developmental studies of blind children: II. *New Outlook for the Blind,* **60**, 179.

WOLTERS, W. H. G., BONEKAMP, A. L. M., and DONCKERWOLTKE, R. (1973). Experience in the development of a haemodialysis center for children. *Journal of Psychosomatic Research,* **17**, 271.

WOOD, A. C., Jr., FRIEDMAN, C. J. and STEISEL, I. M. (1967). Psychosocial factors in phenylketonuria. *American Journal of Orthopsychiatry,* **XXXVII**, 671.

WOODMANSEY, A. C. (1971). Parent guidance. *Developmental Medicine and Child Neurology*, **13**, 243.

WORDEN, D. K. and VIGNOS, P. J., Jr. (1962). Intellectual function in childhood progressive muscular dystrophy. *Pediatrics*, **29**, 968.

WRIGHT, B. (1960). *Physical Disability: A Psychological Approach*. Harper & Row, New York.

WRIGHT, B. (1964). Spread in adjustment to disability. *Bulletin of the Menninger Clinics*, **28**, 198.

WRIGHT, L. (1970). Counselling with parents of chronically ill children. *Postgraduate Medicine*, **47**, 173.

WYLIE, R. C. (1961). *The Self-Concept*. University of Nebraska Press, Lincoln, Nebraska.

WYSOCKI, B. A. and WHITNEY, E. (1965). Body image of crippled as seen in Draw-A-Person test behavior. *Perceptual and Motor Skills*, **21**, 499.

YOUNGHUSBAND, E., BIRCHALL, D., DAVIE, R and KELLMER-PRINGLE, M. L. (1970). Living with handicap — The report of a working party on children with special needs. National Bureau for Co-operation in Child Care, London.

YULE, W. (1973). Epilepsy: Education and Enigma. *Special Education*, **62**, 205.

YULE, W. and RUTTER, M. (1970). Educational aspects of physical disorder. In *Education, Health and Behaviour*, p. 297. (Rutter, M., Tizard, J., Whitmore, K. eds.). Longman, London.

ZAHRAN, H. A. S. (1965). A study of personality differences between blind and sighted children. *British Journal of Educational Psychology*, **35**, 329.

ZEALLEY, A. K., AITKEN, R. C. B. and ROSENTHAL, S. V. (1970). Psychopathology in bronchial asthmatic patients. *Scottish Medical Journal*, **15**, 102.

ZEIDEL, A. (1970). Emotional adjustment of juvenile diabetics and their families. In *Habilitation and Rehabilitation of Juvenile Diabetics. Proceedings of 1st Beilinson Symposium on Juvenile Diabetes*, (Laron, Z. T., ed.). Williams & Wilkins, Baltimore.

ZILLER, R. C., HAGEY, J., SMITH, M. D. and LONG, B. H. (1969). Self-esteem: A self-social construct. *Journal of Consulting and Clinical Psychology*, **33**, 84.

Index

Activity, restrictions of, 136, 157
Acceptance, 180, 189-92
  and adjustment, 25-6, 132-3
  parental, 136
  theoretical implications, 15-16
Adaptation and psychosocial adjustment, 28-9
  to osteogenesis imperfecta, 134
Adjustment,
  and restricted activities, 157
  and severity, 156-7
  basic concepts, 21-3
  definition, 15, 34
  indicators of, 61
  models of, 29-30
  optimal adult, 60-1
Adolescence,
  academic achievement, 66
  psychological consequences during, 64-5
Age at onset, and adjustment,
  of cleft lip or palate, 130
  of haemophilia, 145
  of inappropriate sexual development, 125
  of scoliosis, 127
Ambiguities in congenital deafness, 203
Amputees, adjustment of, 136
Anxiety,
  and congenital heart diseases, 155
  and open-heart surgery, 156
  measures of, 41, 43-4
Arthritis, adjustment studies, 152-4
Asthma, adjustment studies, 147-51
  tests used, 44
Attitudes, and adjustment, 177
  community, 183-5
  parental and family, 178-82
Attributes, intrinsic personality, 30
Autobiographies, of the disabled, 17
  in assessment of adjustment, 132

B
Behaviour, direct observations of, 36
Behavioural modification, 194-5
Bio-psycho-social concept, of adjustment, 176

Bleeding, spontaneous, in haemophilia, 144, 175
Blunting, effect of handicap, 89
Body cathexis, 45
Body image,
  and burns, 126
  and inappropriate sexual development, 125
  and nephrosis, 159
  and orthopaedic disorders, 134
  and skin conditions, 128
  in personality functioning, 45
Briefing, as intervention modality, 203
Brown, Christy, autobiography of, 65
Burns, adjustment studies, 126

C
Camp, summer, for diabetics, 196, 199
Case studies, value of, 138
Carnegie UK Trust, report of, 138
CARIH (Childrens Asthma Research Institute & Hospital), 150
Causality, between illness and adjustment, 32
Central nervous system disorders,
  and scholastic achievement, 97
Cerebral palsy, 37
  adjustment studies, 134
  scholastic achievement, 69
Child rearing, 165
  of diabetics, 142
Chronic illness,
  defined, 90-1
  epidemiology of, 15, 17
  social psychology of, 17
  specific disorders, 18
Cleft lip and palate as cosmetic abnormality, 129
Communication, training for, 207-8
Community, and handicap, 138
  locale for services, 198
Comprehensive health care, 161
Conceptual framework of adjustment, 19
Continuity of relationship, 207-8
Coping,
  and diabetic control, 143
  and surgery, 156

model of adjustment, 27-8
of adolescents with scoliosis, 127
of family, 163
Cosmetic disorders,
adjustment studies, 122-30
Counselling, as intervention, 205-6
of parents, 196-7
Counsellors, family, 95, 201
Co-ordination of services, 184
Criminality as indicator of adjustment, 72
Crisis, psychological, 88
Critical periods and socialization, 140
Cystic fibrosis, adjustment studies, 18, 146-7

D
Daily problems and family life, 139, 165
Deafness, academic achievement, 69
adjustment studies, 18, 39, 116-18
employment level, 83
employment rates, 82-3
Defenses, and adaptive processes, 144
intrapsychic, 29, 127
Denial of disability, 25, 136, 181
Dependency, needs of and adjustment, 132-3
in haemophilia, 146
Development, stage of and adaptation, 89-90
Diabetes, adjustment studies, in childhood, 141-3
in adulthood, 66, 76
Dialysis, renal, 159-60
Didactic model as intervention, 196
Disability, defined, 17, 21
Draw-a-Person test, 54
and heart disease, 155
and Klinefelter's syndrome, 194
and osteogenesis imperfecta, 135
and renal disease, 160
as measure of body image, 134
Dwarfism, academic achievement in, 101
adjustment studies, 127-8
Dying child, 146

E
Education, techniques of, 202-4
Educational achievement and maladjustment, 67
Employment, and intelligence, 84
and severity, 84-5
Endocrine studies and coping with stress, 176
Epidemiological studies, 90

Epilepsy, 17
adjustment studies, 110-13
educational achievement, 99
Extroversion, measures, 42

F
Family,
and blindness, 115
and cerebral palsy, 109
and deafness, 117
and epilepsy, 109
factors affecting adjustment, 162-3
Functioning, Index of, 93
impact of disease, 93, 146, 161, 163, 177
interaction of, 182
isolation of, 183
separation of asthmatics, 150
Family climate, Index of, 119
Fathers, role of, 154
Functioning, psychosocial, 29-30

G
Geographic factors and family problems, 138
Group therapy, 110, 187, 195-6
mothers of burned children, 126
Guilt, parental, 159
and cystic fibrosis, 189
and haemophilia, 180

H
Haemophilia, 17, 37
and academic achievement, 102
adjustment studies, 143-6
Handicap, defined, 22
Health services, planning for, 16
Heart disease, adjustment studies, 154-158
Hospital admissions, indications for, 198

I
Illness behaviour, 28
Impact on family, 163-4
(see also family, impact of disease)
Impairment, defined, 21
Information, techniques of, 202
about heart disease, 156
Intelligence, and blindness, 115
and osteogenesis imperfecta, 135
effect of illness, 103-6
Intervention,
during adolescence, 64
location of, 197-9

INDEX 243

objectives of, 189
preventive, 16-18
purveyors of, 200-2
recipients of, 186
techniques of, 187, 192-9
therapeutic, 31
timing of, 90
Interviews, clinical, as assessment measure, 57
Isle of Wight Survey, 57
  academic achievement, 68, 98
  and deafness, 116
  and epilepsy, 98
  psychiatric disorder, 93

K

Kidney disease, adjustment studies of, 158-61
  (see also nephrosis, renal disease, dialysis)
Klinefelter's syndrome, and behaviour, and criminality, 72
  (see also chromosome disorders, XXY syndrome)
Knowledge of diabetes and control, 143

L

Life space as somatopsychological concept, 24
Locomotor disorders, adjustment studies of, 131-40
  defined, 131

M

MMPI as indicator of adult adjustment, 75-7
Maladjustment, psychosocial, 16
  (see also adjustment, acceptance, adaptation)
Marginality, and adjustment, 76
  in arthritis, 153
  in partial blindness, 114
  in partial deafness, 114, 118
  in thalidomide syndrome, 116
Marital stability as indicator of adult adjustment, 73
Maternal attitudes and heart disease, 157
Measures of adjustment, 34-5
Meningomyelocele and intelligence, 105
Mothers, emotional disturbances of, 142
Muscular dystrophy and intelligence, 104-5
Myopia, academic achievement of, 100

N

National Survey of Health and Development,
  academic achievement of, 67, 100
  1946 Cohort, 81, 91, 100, 137
  1958 Cohort, 39, 100
Nature-nurture controversy, 30, 120
Nature of illness, 169-73
Nephrosis, adjustment studies, 159
Neuroticism, measures of, 42
Newson, John and Elizabeth, questionnaire, 165
Normality, concept of, 22-3
  of osteogenesis imperfecta, 135
Nursery programmes, 199

O

Obesity, body image in, 45
  college acceptance, 71
Observations of behaviour, 38
Ombudsman, doctor as, 200
Optimism, role of, 191
Osteogenesis imperfecta, adjustment studies of, 134-5
Overcompensation, 26

P

Parent education, hospital-based, 198
Parental acceptance and adjustment, 136
Parental assessment of abilities, 108
Parental attitudes,
  general importance of, 178
  to cleft palate, 129
  to physical handicap, 138
Parental reactions to facial deformities, 125
Parental relations, and diabetic adjustment, 142
  and adjustment of haemophiliacs, 144
Parents as members of rehabilitation team, 129, 196
Peer ratings, as measure of adjustment, 39
Personal reaction, to disability, 174-5
Personality, inventories of, 42-4
  super-stable, 192
Physical disability and academic achievement, 102
Physical procedures, as intervention, 194
  in adjustment to heart disease, 157, 158
Poliomyelitis, adjustment studies of, 43

Practical provisions as intervention, 208-209
Prejudice, 184
   and marriage rates, 73
   to cosmetic abnormalities, 123
   to obese college applicants, 71
   to the deaf in employment, 83
Prematurity and educational achievement, 101
Primary physician, role of, 161, 204
Projective measures as measure of adjustment, 53-5
Psychiatric disorder, during adolescence, 64
   during adulthood, 78
   during childhood, 93
   in deaf children, 116
Psychologic disorders, and cerebral palsy, 107-8
   and CNS disorders, 106
   and poliomyelitis, 106-7
   as indicators of adjustment, 74
Psychosomatic aetiology, and asthma, 147
   and rheumatoid arthritis, 152
Psychotherapy, brief, 195
   and psychologic test results, 161

Q
Q-sort technique, as measure of adjustment, 60
   as measure of self-perception, 47

R
Rating scales, as indicators of adjustment, 38-9
Reaction patterns of disabled, 25-6
Research, implementation of, 18
   nature of, 16
   summary of, 16-17
Residential schooling, 199
   and deafness, 119-20
   and employment, 83
Restitution-avoidance dichotomy, 137
Restrictions, activity, 135
   theoretical significance, 130
Rheumatic fever, adult adjustment, 77-8
Risk level, amount of intervention, 187
   factors related, 88
Rochester studies of chronic illness, 40, 49, 160
Rorschach test, in haemophilia, 145

S
Scholastic achievement,
   and family factors, 98
   attitude of teachers, 110
   as indirect indicator of adjustment, 95
   effect of absences, 103
   of children with kidney disease, 160
   of children with non-CNS disorders, 101-2
Scoliosis, adjustment studies of, 126
Sears, Macoby and Levin, interview guide, 166
Self-concept, evaluation of, 26
   formation of, 24
   in dialysis or transplantation, 160
   in heart disease, 155
   model of, 24
   scales of, 45, 48
Self-derogation and adjustment, 46-7
Self-description of disabled, 140
Self-ideal discrepancy, measures of, 43, 47
Self-image, and orthopaedic disorders, 140
   measures of, 45
   of deaf child, 119
   role of, 181
   (see also body image)
Self-social personality theory, constructs test, 52
Semantic differential technique,
   and asthma, 150
   and cleft palate, 130
   and locomotor disorder, 133
Sensory disorders, adjustment studies of, 113-22
   effect on cognitive development, 114-115
Services, allocation of, 188
Severity, and adjustment, 157, 133
   and employment, 84
Sex difference, and adult adjustment, 75, 77
   and employment, 83
   and intelligence, 104
   in diabetes, behavioural symptoms of, 142
   in self-descriptions, 140
'Significant others' in response to disability, 30
Skin conditions, adjustment studies of, 128
   (see also cosmetic disorders)
Social factors, and adjustment,

in cosmetic abnormalities, 124
in epilepsy, 111
Social integration of disabled, 185
Social sensitivity and adjustment, 136
Social workers, intervention by, 201
Socialization of young handicapped, 140
Sociometry, methods, 40
  modified for amputees, 139
Sociopsychological consequences of disability, 89
Somatopsychology, and locomotor disorders, 131
  of disabilities, 24, 33, 76
Special education, advantages of, 67
  and employment of the deaf, 83
  and physically handicapped, 137
  and sensory disorders, 113
  crippled children's school, 69
  referral criteria, 184
  residential schools, 67
  standards of instruction, 96
Speech disorders, adjustment studies of, 121-2
  use of sociometric measures, 40, 122
Spread, phenomenon of, 22, 26
  and repercussions of therapy, 195
Squints, academic achievement, 100
Stature, deviations of, as cosmetic abnormality, 127
Stereotyping, of asthmatic child, 148
  phenomenon of, 26
Stigma, and blind stereotyped activity, 114
  and speech disorders, 121
Subjective measures as indicators of adjustment, 40

Suicide, and diabetes, 67
  as indirect indicator of adjustment during adolescence, 66
Symptomatic concordance, principle of, 192
Systemic disorders, adjustment studies of, 141-61

T

Teachers' attitudes, 124
Team approach, co-ordinated, 153, 198
Technical expertise, access to, 204
Thalidomide, adjustment studies of, 133
  deformities due to, 17
  effects on mothering, 165-6
Therapist, orientation of, 182-3
Timing of intervention, 190, 203
Transplantation, renal, 158
Treatment, consequences of, 77
Tutoring as therapeutic intervention, 195

V

Ventilation as therapeutic intervention, 195
Visibility of disorder, 123, 140
Vision, disturbances of and educational achievement, 100
  (see also blindness)
Vocational achievement as indicator of adjustment, 81
Vulnerable child syndrome, 26

W

Withdrawal as psychological defense, 25
  (see also denial)

NO LONGER THE PROPERTY OF THE UNIVERSITY OF R. I. LIBRARY